T0040318

Advanced Praise for *Bioenergy Healing*

"Outstanding exploration of a scientist turned healer's experience in working with patients to utilize the energy that fills the universe. This short volume teaches the reader how to cut to the core of health issues and live happily and healthily. It gets rid of the crutch mentality, where drugs and surgery are the only healing techniques and draws on the concepts of traditional medicine globally. Csongor Daniel uses the subtle methods of mind, body and spirit for healing and works with a clean environment, internally and externally."

—Diane Wolff
Author

"In just 238 short pages Csongor eloquently yet simply explains that we all have the potential to heal. We are all energetic beings, and everything is energy. These are not easy concepts for most of us to accept or understand. Yet through undeniable scientific data, relating to our personal experiences and using his own often humorous stories, Csongor leaves you with no doubt that we all have the innate ability to heal simply using energy.

"What's more, Csongor uses a quarter century of his own experience and the teachings he received from his Master to reveal a system of healing that will forever change the way you experience and understand how we create disease in the body, how the body heals, and how we can heal each other."

—Stephen Edwards
Author, Speaker

"I have training in the Domancic bioenergy healing method, personal bioenergy healing experience with Csongor Daniel, and mentoring experience with him as well. It is a privilege to share my impressions of his latest book. First and foremost, it is a nicely distilled documentation of bioenergy theory, exercises, and practice. It is therefore quite useful to apprentice and novice energy healers. Experienced bioenergy healers will find utility in the compendium of protocols in the book. As a psychotherapist who is blending bioenergy with psychotherapy, I am appreciative of the case studies detailing how bioenergy treatments are integrated with other modalities. Csongor's writing style is easy to read. He invites the reader along at a nice but effective pace. It's a worthy read for anyone interested in bioenergy healing."

—Gregory Boyce, M.A.
Author, *No More Drama: A Practical Guide to Healthy Relationships*

"Csongor Daniel has the most amazing balanced energy of anyone I've ever met. He has the ability to then use this incredible talent for the good of others. Not only have I watched him heal with his abilities, I've been a recipient of his work. I credit Csongor with giving my life back to me when I thought fibromyalgia and chronic fatigue had reduced my life to that of an invalid. I always refer clients to him with the greatest of confidence. I also teach my Intuitive Arts students his process of learning to 'see,' 'feel,' and 'use' energy directly from his book, *Bioenergy: A Healing for the 21st Century*. He truly is a gift to all of us."

—Betty McCormack,
Master Practitioner of Intuitive Arts

Bioenergy Healing

Simple Techniques for Reducing
Pain and Restoring Health through
Energetic Healing

Csongor Daniel

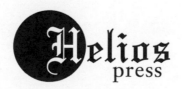

Copyright © 2016 by Csongor Daniel

All rights reserved. No part of this book may be reproduced in any manner without the express written consent of the publisher, except in the case of brief excerpts in critical reviews or articles. All inquiries should be addressed to Helios Press, 307 West 36th Street, 11th Floor, New York, NY 10018.

Helios books may be purchased in bulk at special discounts for sales promotion, corporate gifts, fund-raising, or educational purposes. Special editions can also be created to specifications. For details, contact the Special Sales Department, Skyhorse Publishing, 307 West 36th Street, 11th Floor, New York, NY 10018 or info@skyhorsepublishing.com.

Helios Press is an imprint of Skyhorse Publishing, Inc.®, a Delaware corporation.

Visit our website at www.skyhorsepublishing.com.

10 9 8 7 6 5 4

Library of Congress Cataloging-in-Publication Data is available on file.

Print ISBN: 9781634503914
Ebook ISBN: 9781634508612

Cover design by Jane Sheppard
Cover photo credit: Thinkstock

Printed in China

This book is not intended as a substitute for the medical advice of physicians; the methods discussed are not designed to replace conventional medicine. The reader should regularly consult a physician in matters relating to his/her health and particularly with respect to any symptoms that may require diagnosis or medical attention.

To all who need healing
and
To all who want to help

TABLE OF CONTENTS

Introduction

Fifteen years after publishing my first book, *Biotherapy: A Healing for the 21st Century*, as well as teaching hundreds of lectures and seminars in the United States and internationally, I realized that I could teach anyone to become a healer. Furthermore, I was assured that I could accomplish that in as little as one day. My seminars were enough evidence to back up that conviction. Putting it in writing was the next step. However, as the sentences and pages started piling up, the perfectionist in me wouldn't leave anything out. I wanted to give the beginner healer all the necessary intellectual and practical knowledge to not only help themselves, but to become proficient in healing anyone needing help. Instead of the target 50 pages—which any person could have read in a day—the book just kept growing and eventually ended up the size you are holding now.

Bioenergy healing can truly be learned as fast as you can read; however, it takes a lot of practice and a lifetime of experience to perfect. By relating my own knowledge and experiences, I hope I was able to cut that time shorter for you. Whether you wish to help yourself, your family members, your friends, or thousands of strangers, I trust *Bioenergy Healing* will aid you in that quest. Moreover, if I help you to heal only one person in your lifetime, all my work will be well worth it.

Thank you for your interest in *Bioenergy Healing* and your noble desire to heal others.

1.

You Too Can Be a Healer: You *Are* a Healer

Chances are, if you picked up this book, you already believe that you can heal. However, even if you have no such ambitions, you automatically became a healer the moment you were born.

Think about it: when you cut yourself, is it the bandage that stops the bleeding? Of course not! It is your body's incredible ability to repair itself. The bandage just keeps the wound (and your clothes) clean and prevents further injury.

When you have a cold, is it the ibuprofen, or the echinacea, or the extra vitamin C that heals you? Those things surely make your life less miserable, but they don't heal you; they just assist you. It is again your body that does it.

This is nothing new. It happens to animals and plants as well. Every living creature has the ability—the mechanism—to repair itself in one way or another.

Sometimes we do need a little boost in the form of medicine or surgery, but many times something as simple as a hug will do. Think again: when your children get hurt, what do you do? You pick them up, hug them, and kiss or stroke the painful spot, right? Sure, there is quite a psychological factor helping to stop the pain, but what you don't realize is that there is a tremendous amount of energy exchanging between you and your child at that moment. Did they need medicine or surgery to stop the pain? No. It was your embrace alone that did the trick.

What do you feel when you hug someone? Warmth? Tingling? Some trembling even? Either way, it is a pleasant feeling accompanied by a significant energy-mingle between two huggers.

Most of the preceding examples happen without us noticing the actual energy. It is similar to walking down the street and feeling that there is someone behind us—which we usually confirm by turning around and indeed finding someone there. We don't think about any energy at the time; we just have a "feeling."

Do you know the game where you stare at someone's temple in the movie theatre until they turn around? Same thing—it is the energy they will eventually feel, but they will turn around on a whim, not because they think that a particular force field is disturbing their peace.

This energy is everywhere and literally *is* everything. It travels any distance in a speck of time. How many times have you thought of someone just to hear the phone ring a moment later with that person on the other line? I bet this thought put a smile on your face, right? Indeed, it happens to all of us. You may even have a special person (or a few people) that it happens with more often than with others. Sharing this connection with your friends or loved ones is quite fun, isn't it? I have an aunt with whom this connection is so strong that it became a competition. Just the thought of her will make me leap for the phone, because I know her call is coming. I try to beat her to it and call first. To which she would say: "Wow, I was just about to call you! You beat me again!" Of course, this goes the other way round quite often as well.

My strongest connection is with my girlfriend, with whom I don't even have to set up a time to talk. It is just a feeling that makes me pick up a phone and call her. Quite often I get the answer after the very first ring: "You are a sage!" Again, it goes both ways.

Does this mean that we are all psychics? In a way: yes. We all have abilities beyond our imagination. We call them psychic powers or other metaphysical names only because we don't have any firm scientific explanations for them—or at least we don't know of them in our everyday lives. The mass media doesn't handle healing and other "psychic phenomena" in a scientific manner. Rather, they are presented in sensationalized or preposterous ways, as reporters search for the miracles in them or simply try to ridicule them.

Think of some old "facts": The sun revolves around the earth; the earth is flat; nothing heavier than air will ever fly; everything there is to know has already been invented; and so on. Every generation needs an open mind—including ours.

In reality, we all have the ability to sense one another whether we are close by or separated by great distances. We just don't utilize that ability enough. It is easier to open our mouths and talk. Convenience dictates picking up the phone or sending a message. It is common knowledge that we use a very small amount of our brain capacity (and manage to reduce even that within a lifetime). If we could use more or most of it, who knows where we could be? Maybe we would talk telepathically or even hover around defying gravity! We certainly would be able to control our bodies better in order to keep them healthy. Why not do it now?

I ask at the beginning of each lecture and seminar: "What is the most important thing in your life?" After the usual responses are out of the way (kids, grandkids, husband, wife, or a valued animal or asset), eventually everyone comes to the same conclusion: it is your health. Without it you couldn't take care of your loved ones and the other important things in your life. It is directly or indirectly the tool that enables you to achieve everything you want in life.

The follow-up question: how much *time* do you spend every day on the most important thing in your life? This is when most people start turning their heads and avoiding eye contact.

Sure, we sleep, brush our teeth, and do other things every day that directly affect our health, but do we really consciously *think* about our health every day? Some of us may, but most people don't. Blindly following outdated health doctrines does not help. For instance, our conscience may be clear about drinking milk because the ad said: "It does a body good!" But does it really? Have you checked lately? Have you googled it yet?

Our health is the most precious thing we have in our lifetime. Just ask anyone—rich or poor, young or old—who has lost it! The richest man lying on his death bed would give anything in order to be healthy again. Anything. That is the bottom line.

However, when we are healthy, we do take it for granted. Just think of how many times you have stuffed your face with fast food, sugary carbonated drinks, or calories of questionable origins! Our health doesn't come cheap. We have to maintain it. We have to nourish it. We have to guard it.

At the risk of going on a rant here, the bottom line is this: you and only you are responsible for your own health and you can't expect others to do it for you. You certainly can't blame others—especially not your TV set—if things go sour. Accept that the food and medical industries are primarily businesses with a need for profit. You come in second. Thankfully, nowadays you don't have to spend hours in the library searching through literature in order to find answers to your health questions. Sit down by your computer, and in mere minutes, you will have your answers. I just wanted to wake up your curiosity and give you a little kick in the butt.

I certainly can't change everything about you or anyone else. It would be impossible. However, if I can help you even a little bit and give you directions on how to improve your health and well-being—furthermore, how to heal others—I have made a difference in this world. I did my part by writing down all my healing knowledge. Now it is up to you to read it and implement it. This book is truly dedicated to teaching you to become a healer as fast as you can read—in as little as a few days!

2.
Everything Is Energy

If you look at the human body, it appears to be solid—flexible yes, but still solid. Yet, we know that roughly 70 percent of the body is water (with variations, depending on one's age). Can you hear that water splashing around? Of course not because it is contained in trillions of tiny little balloons called cells. Let's magnify an individual cell—or better yet: an individual drop of water. We will find that it is made of molecules. These also resemble balloons, and are filled with gases: hydrogen and oxygen. Now, if we could go deeper into them, at higher magnification, we would find atoms—the tiniest particles that make up the entire universe.

Let's review the atom, in case you skipped your quantum physics class. When you think of atomic structure, you may compare it to the solar system: in the middle of the atom, you have the nucleus (like the sun in the middle of the solar system). Surrounded by electrons (like the planets around the sun) traveling at a certain distance from the middle, never drifting away or collapsing into the center. The real key to understanding energy is the actual distance between the nucleus (or the sun) and the electrons (or planets). For a moment, don't think of the model of the solar system sitting on the teacher's desk that you remember from school. That was only a visual aid that has nothing to do with accuracy. The real model would be impossible to contain in any school facility. The actual distances are just mind-boggling: If we could shrink the sun to the size of a pea, Pluto (sorry, Pluto, for losing your planetary status, but it is the last rock in our solar system) would be a mile and a half away, and it would be the size of a bacterium! Yet, they still stay together in their predetermined path, held together by this invisible force we call gravity.

The actual atomic structure is even more unbelievable. If we could magnify the nucleus (which is positively charged) to be the size of a pin head and put it in the middle of a stadium, the closest electron (which is negatively charged) would be outside the bleachers! Moreover, the weight of the entire stadium (or atom in this case) would be contained in that single nucleus! Now imagine the tiny electron as only a speck of dust (if even that) traveling around the stadium at such breakneck speed that you would never be able to actually point it out. It would cover any spot in the stadium at any given moment, giving it the appearance of a full ball. Yes, to an outsider, the atom would appear to be a ball. However, we know that it is not. Most of that atom is just the energy holding things together; 99.9999999999 percent (give or take a few nines) of the atom is just empty space, like the universe itself. As in the universe, there are some distant "stars" in the atom as well, called quarks, as well as other tiny "particles," but they are not important for the purposes of our visualization.

Now, if you take one of these near empty stadiums and find another nearly empty stadium and then another mega zillion of these, you will end up with a human body. We do appear solid, but we know that deep down we are made of mostly nothing—99.9999999999 percent of our bodies is empty space, to be more accurate. We are primarily pure energy.

We also know that our bodies are electromagnetic in nature. Our nerves transfer electromagnetic signals all day long. Our heartbeat is regulated by electric current, and our hearts transfer an electrical charge to the blood cells as they travel through. Not to mention our electromagnetic brain activity. As a matter of fact, we can measure everything in our bodies in the same way that we can measure electrical current in a radio or TV set: we have amps, ohms, volts, and so on.

As with power lines that are surrounded by an electromagnetic field as long as there is current, our bodies are surrounded by an electromagnetic field as well. In the power lines, the field can be measured, and it can be mathematically accounted for. The human body is a bit more delicate and complex than that. It would be quite difficult to get an accurate reading, and quantifying it would be nearly impossible. There are ways to photograph the field around us, but those are still not precise enough. Kirlian photography has been around since the 1930s and has shown mixed results. It is possible to take pictures of the aura around your hand or a leaf or various other objects or body parts. However, the photo can't give a precise measurement of the energy field. There are Kirlian machines that will depict what the aura around your head may look like in real time, but those, again, are just electromagnetic connections read off your

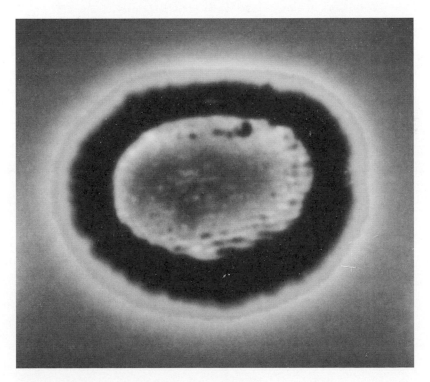

Kirlian photo of the author's right middle finger at rest (nice and even)

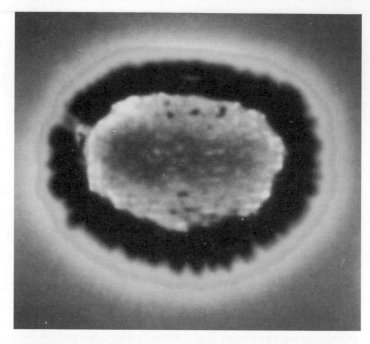

Same finger during negative thoughts (note how it is broken up)

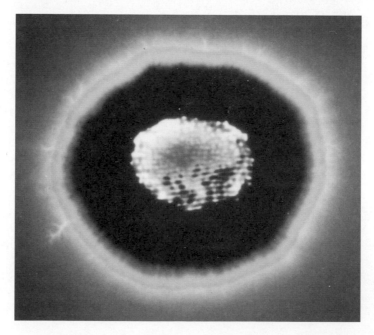

Same finger during healing (note the size and intensity)

hand (through a conductive plate) and subsequently transformed in a computer to a picture around your head. They are great for new age expos, but not good enough for modern medical diagnoses.

Contemporary medicine still has the best diagnostic methods. Unfortunately, it separates the mind from the body (or the electromagnetic from the physical) and doesn't look at the human being as a whole. It is important to realize that, as with all things in the universe, our energy tries to stay in a certain balance, as depicted in the t'ai chi symbol, a.k.a. the yin and yang. We learned that the human energy field itself is connected to every aspect of our being: mind, body, spirit, emotions, and whatnot. Balancing the energy will thus affect every part. Many times I had clients with certain physical problems, and they reported improvements in their mental and emotional lives, too. Vice versa as well. Balancing produces positive side effects.

According to Chinese philosophy, everything is comprised of opposites: male–female, hot–cold, mountain–valley, fire–water, and so forth. There is always a little bit of one in the other. However, one cannot overtake the other—that would mean the end of them both, or death.

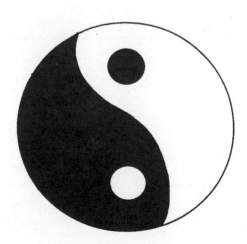

Our universe as well as our energy system tries to stay in infinite balance. In the case of an inanimate object—for instance, a plastic chair (which, mind you, is also made of energy)—this balance is persistent until the moment we burn that chair or disintegrate it in another fashion. Our bodies are quite different. Our energy changes all the time, virtually every moment of our lives. It depends on many factors, such as nutrition, environment, the people around us, our thoughts, and so forth. It is practically impossible to keep it balanced for long periods of time, yet we don't necessarily become ill every time it goes out of the equilibrium. The problems start when we have parts of the energy out of balance for longer periods of time. Most illnesses actually show up first in the energy field and only later in the body. As a general rule, the healthy aura is always smooth and even at an approximate distance of an arm's length from the body. We may feel imbalances in parts of it even when the person feels perfectly healthy—that again is because the problems will show in the field before they show in the body. Thus, it is sometimes possible to predict a problem before it happens. Naturally, this doesn't apply to injuries and violent acts with baseball bats, bullets, and such.

The ultimate goal is to stay as close to the balance as possible, at any given moment in our lives.

3.
The Healthy Aura

O ur energy field is described and referred to in many ways in various languages and at different times in history: Chi (China), Ki (Japan), Bioenergy (Russia, Europe), Animal Magnetism (Austria, late 1700s–1800s via Franz Mesmer's experiments), Spiritus (old Rome), Prana (India), Mana, Bioplasma, Pneuma, Vital fluid, Odic force, Orgone . . . and Aura. Whatever we call it, it is the same thing.

There also are many different healing methods that deal with that same thing: Therapeutic Touch (TT), Healing Touch, Acupuncture, Acupressure, Reiki, QiGong, Quantum Touch, Esoteric Healing, Magnetic Healing, Crystal Healing, Pranic Healing, and of course Bioenergy Healing, or Biotherapy. It is impossible to list them all, since there are new methods popping up virtually every day. However, they all deal with the same energy, just in different ways. I liken it to cars. They all have four wheels, and they all take you places; some of them just do it faster and fancier than others. I like to think of Biotherapy (or Bioenergy Healing) as the Ferrari of energy healing. It is one of the fastest and most effective methods out there.

The healthy energy field is smooth and even around the whole body extending to an approximate distance of an arm's length. It forms a sort of egg-shaped shield around us, similar to the protective energy shield around the starship Enterprise, just wider.

The human aura has distinguishable layers, with the thinnest running just millimeters around the skin. The layers are connected to the chakras—energy centers along the midline of the body.

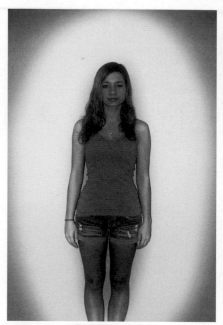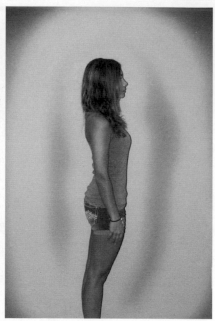

Healthy energy field

There are seven main chakras and twenty-one secondary ones, although each fingertip and toe-tip has one as well. Each chakra is connected to corresponding areas of the body including internal organs. Some authors propose there are nine main chakras while others count eleven, but for our purposes, the different numbers are not so important. We do affect them greatly in the healing process; however, it is not crucial to know all about them in order to heal.

The chakras—if we could see them—would look like small funnels or tornadoes coming out of the body. What we do see—after the first training session—is brightness in the areas where they are supposed to be.

The healthy chakra is smooth, straight, and even. If there is a problem it is indicated by a rough, bent, or uneven shape. Regardless of whether we can see chakras or not, bioenergy healing will affect them in a positive way and it will affect all of them, since our healing method concentrates on the whole being as one unit.

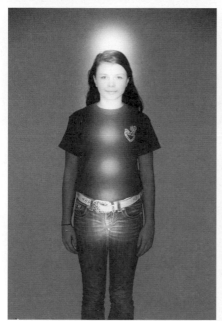
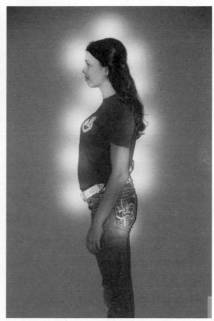

Main chakras

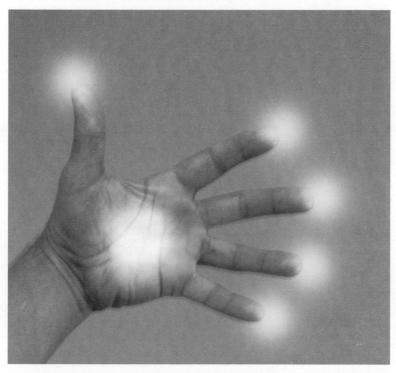

Secondary chakras of the hand

The goal of the healthy energy field is to stay balanced and smooth under all circumstances. It does change every moment of our lives, but it tends to go back to that balance as soon as possible. For instance, if someone cuts you off on the road while driving, the energy increases all around you for a quick speck of time (part of the fight-or-flight response), followed by a period of low energy—a result of the anger, fright, or anguish you may experience. The length of this time period depends on your personality: you may let it go within seconds, or you may carry it as low energy all day long. In this case, the imbalance is not limited to just one area, but spreads throughout the whole energy field. This would result in a weaker immune system and less protection to your body in general. However, in most instances, it is forgotten quickly, and your energy resumes the usual balance. The same scenario would occur in the case of eating or drinking something unhealthy—the energy would return to balance after full digestion.

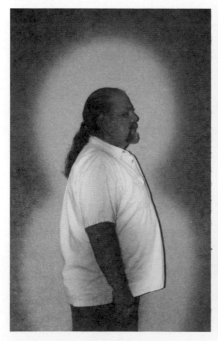 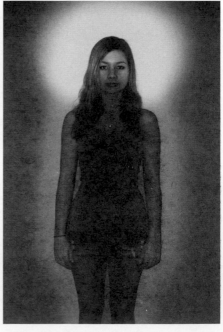

Aura indicating lung imbalance   Aura indicating excess of energy
                                   around head

In the opposite scenario, happy thoughts make the field much wider and stronger as long as the thoughts last. Healthy food and beverages do the same. We will discuss this in more detail later on.

The real problems start (or are indicated) when part of the field is out of balance for a longer period of time. For instance, less energy around the lungs would be the indication of either asthma, bronchitis, or other lung problems, or the by-product of smoking.

On the other hand, excess energy in a small area of the aura is also an indication of a problem, usually associated with pain, inflammation, hyperactivity, and similar overabundances of sensation; such is the case with headaches.

In the case of headaches, the modern response is to take a few painkillers and numb the pain. There are many other options, though, including a quick bioenergy treatment. It takes me about two minutes to stop a headache, even without touching the person. A novice healer may take five to ten minutes—which is still faster than Tylenol!

Most new students ask me the same questions: "Will I be able to do that?" "Can anyone do that?" "Do I have to be gifted to do biotherapy?"

The answer is simple. Just like anything else in the world, anyone can do this to a certain degree. We can all learn to play basketball, right? However—even though I consider myself a good player—I know I will never slam-dunk like Michael Jordan. I have a certain height limitation that prevents me from doing that. We can all learn to play the piano, but again, I will never play like Liszt or Chopin. The bottom line is that we can all do anything we want. However, we are better in certain things than in others. The same goes with bioenergy healing. You will find your full potential as you learn and practice.

4.

The (Energetic) Reasons for Illness

As we know, everything is energy; thus everything vibrates at a certain frequency. When you listen to your car radio and travel far from the radio station, eventually another similar frequency interferes and distorts your reception. The same happens when you listen to music and someone with a louder stereo passes by. In similar fashion, our energy field gets disrupted by other sources of vibration—and there are many.

Source

Electromagnetic fields: Since we are of electromagnetic nature, other electromagnetic fields may disrupt this balance. These could be TV sets, computers, microwave ovens, cell phones, fluorescent light, power lines, and so on. Anything in our vicinity will change our field. The influence depends on the strength of the source. For instance, electrical power lines above the house will disrupt the bioenergy more than an alarm clock radio by our bedside. A study in Britain concluded that a ten-minute conversation on the cell phone will disrupt the bioenergy for almost a week! In similar fashion, fluorescent lights don't give off the full spectrum of light; plus, they vibrate at a level our eyes can barely notice, just enough to mess with our bioenergy.

Solution

What can we do to protect ourselves? Well, aside from moving to a remote mountain location where only some radio waves would disrupt our peace, we will always be a target for electromagnetic radiation. Most of us have already developed a certain electromagnetic immune response, where our energy became stronger and replenishes itself faster due to everyday "training." However, we do need to take certain precautions, such as talking as little as possible on cell phones, and when we do, using earpieces instead of holding the radiation source to our heads. We can sit far from the TV set or have a glass of water between us and the set (water sucks in energy, whether it is positive or negative). Sit far from the computer screen or limit time on the computer. Keep the alarm clock far from your head. Move away from the power lines. . . .

Source

Food: We are what we eat, right? Just as we won't put diesel in our gasoline-burning cars because it will destroy the engine, we shouldn't put bad fuel in our own bodies either. We cannot ignore the signs. On a pack of cigarettes, it says that if we smoke it, it will kill us. Unfortunately, we don't have these warning signs on food packages, so we have to be diligent in finding the right foods ourselves. Simply take more time researching, reading labels, and learning about the ingredients that you can't pronounce. In fact, here's a good guideline: if you can't pronounce it, don't eat it! You may have noticed that most grocery stores have a health food aisle. What is the rest of the store then?! We need to educate ourselves in order to guard our health.

Just a little nutritional wake-up call: Besides the right amount of carbohydrates, fats, and protein from natural, organic, wholesome foods, your body needs at least 90 different nutrients a day—more than 60 minerals, 16 vitamins, 13 amino acids, and three fatty acids, give or take. How many do you get daily? Of course, it would be impossible to account for everything in our food, but you do have to strive for excellence. It is sad to see that most of the country (and the world) is giving in to the fast-paced lifestyle that includes fast food and tons of sugar. As a matter of fact, at this moment, two thirds of the population of the United States is overweight while almost a third is outright obese!

Your blood's natural pH is 7.365. Your entire body is supposed to be slightly alkaline at all times. This is where it functions properly. Only your stomach and large intestines are acidic. However, thanks to the typical Western diet, most people are becoming more and more acidic. All illness, disease, cancer, bacteria, virus, inflammation, arthritis, and other undesirable conditions thrive in an acidic environment (there are some very rare exceptions). When eating acidic foods, your body tries to protect its alkalinity in several ways. It will try to attach the acid to fat and pull it away from the internal organs (that part is quite visible!), or it will try to neutralize the acid with minerals, such as calcium, magnesium, potassium, and such. If you don't have enough of those in your diet, it will pull the same minerals out of your bones, eventually causing osteoporosis, arthritis, inflammation, and such.

Solution

Please read up on this subject as well. With the proper diet, not only can you ward off most illnesses while becoming alkaline and healthy, but your body will drop fat as a side effect, and you will truly feel like a million dollars!

If you are not looking for a lifestyle change, the least you can do is stay away from humankind's greatest enemy: processed sugar. The latest studies suggest that it is the main ingredient at the source of every illness and disease, including cancer and Alzheimer's disease. In fact, you may want to stay away from all processed carbohydrates if you want to lead a healthy life. Nothing good can be found in treated, bleached flour or rice, or any other grains for that matter.

Limit all animal food sources to the minimum, and increase live green vegetables to the maximum . . . do your homework!

Source

Water: In the process of becoming healthy, you should also pay attention to what you drink. Your body was made to process calories from food—not from drinks. Food stays in your stomach for a very long time—hours. Liquids leave the stomach within fifteen or so minutes. If those liquids contain any sugar, it will reach the blood much faster than it would from food, which has to break down slowly to that level. The quick load of sugar in the body requires a panicky insulin production from your pancreas, which not only gets exhausted in the process, but continues doing so until there is no more sugar in the system. Suddenly, the body will find itself in need of sugar—now because of the overabundance of insulin. That's when you experience the "sugar low." Another quick swig of the carbonated sugary drink temporarily fixes the problem, but it just leads to the same vicious cycle.

Drinking diet soda is not a solution—it will just make things worse. By now, your body has learned to respond to the sweetness in the mouth. Before the sweet stuff even reaches the stomach, the pancreas gets into insulin production mode, not knowing that there really isn't any sugar coming. You automatically put yourself into the low sugar mode that makes you hungry. It is quite counterproductive, isn't it? Not to mention that most diet drinks are sweetened with aspartame, which is a derivative of wood alcohol (methyl alcohol), which in the body breaks down into formaldehyde and further into formic acid, which contributes to acidosis and all of its related problems.

Solution

So what can you drink? Since pure glacier milk (highly alkaline and mineral-rich water) is not readily available to all of us, try mineral water, regular spring water, or any filtered water clear of pollutants and chemicals. Do your research, and you will find good sources of water filters, alkalizers, ionizers, and such. Litmus paper is cheap and excellent for checking your water's alkalinity. Green tea and other herbal teas are good, as well as certain super greens and other green powdered water additives. Let your taste buds experience foods. Relax them when you drink. You will notice minute differences even in the taste of various types of water. Energize the water yourself! It can't be healthier than that. Read up on it at the end of this book.

Source

Geopathic zones or geopathic stress: These are mostly underground areas where, for certain reasons, the energy is disrupted and negatively affects your energy field. These areas may not be too dangerous, but spending a lot of time above them will eventually take its toll. If you sleep above a geopathic zone for many years, it will slowly drain your energy, and you may become vulnerable to serious disease. Some people are sensitive to those areas, which may result in sleeping problems, getting up tired, having headaches, and so on. Working or studying in those areas will result in more tiredness, lack of concentration, and general lethargy.

Solution

If you suspect that you live above a cave or cavern, underground water, or other source of geopathic stress, the best solution is to either move away or at least move your bed to a safe location. There are some sophisticated instruments that can measure and find these locations; however, they may not be available to you. Trained dowsers may be a better solution. Dowsers are people who raised their sensitivity level using such instruments as dowsing rods or pendulums, and they usually search for water, oil, and other underground goods, including treasure. Many are specialized in finding geopathic zones. This is another science that most people can learn, including you! Learn the fastest way to dowse from: *Biotherapy: A Healing for the 21*st *Century* by yours truly.

If you can't move, the cheapest solution to counter the negative radiation would be to repel it by some metal (mostly copper) rods or plates placed under your bed or work station. Again, do diligent research!

There are many instruments, gadgets, and gizmos that neutralize most harmful radiation (including electromagnetic fields and geopathic stress), such as Q-link, Teslar, Tachyon, and others—with more or less success. New technologies appear every day, so again: research. Read up on dowsing at the end of this book . . .

Source

Cosmic radiation: There is not much we can do about this one, but we have to mention it. There are many types of cosmic rays that hit us all the time, day and night. Gamma rays, X-rays, protons, and similar energy types that originate mostly outside the solar system, are divided into primary and secondary rays. The secondary are the ones that penetrate the earth's magnetic field and may be harmful to us whether on the ground or in an airplane. Most of us are quite resistant to these radiations since we have been bombarded by them since birth. Some radiation can penetrate the earth and bounce back, picking up some negative energy from sources such as geopathic zones and eventually hitting us with slightly more negativity than on the way down. Note that by "negativity" or "negative energy," we don't mean "minus"; rather, we mean the negative influence on our energy.

Solution

Relax, it is not that bad. However, if you are worried, this can also be tackled with dowsing.

Source

Environment: Your energy will be greatly affected by your surroundings. I don't think we have to talk much about this one. Where do you feel better—in downtown Beijing during the smog alerts or on a clean Florida beach? Downtown Detroit or the Smoky Mountains? In the middle of the Sahara or Hawaii? You get my drift.

Solution

Find a clean environment where you feel good, and stick to it!

Source

Weather: We do feel the changes in weather, right? A nice, sunny spring day will certainly affect us in a better way than a dreary, rainy fall day. The atmospheric pressure goes unnoticed by some people while others feel it tremendously.

Solution

There is not much we can do about it. However, it is crucial to know that it will affect some people; thus, it will affect the outcome of their treatments.

Source

Other people: Birds of a feather? We all have family and friends that we spend time with. How do you feel in their presence? Good friends and close family literally breathe fresh energy into your system. You know the feeling when a happy-go-lucky friend of yours shows up with a great smile. It is catchy, isn't it? You can just feel their energy as a huge bubble around them making your energy open up and smile. On the other hand, you may also have one (or more) of those friends or family members who are constant downers. They are always in a bad mood, complaining and negative, even when things are perfectly alright. How do you feel in their presence? They "drain" your energy, right? It is not just in your head; people do influence your energy greatly. Any time you are less than an arm's length from a person, you are definitely in their energy and under their influence. This distance is proportionate to the person's energy field and at times can go to practically infinity. Think of a rock star on a stage influencing thousands of people all at the same time. The negative influence can also be just as big. Prolonged exposure to the "negative" people will eventually drain your energy to very low levels, where the resultant decrease in your immunity may lead to illness.

Solution

We know that we can't choose family, but we can certainly choose friends. If you feel that someone is draining your energy, you have to do something about it. Either talk it over with that person, or spend less or no time with them. I know this sounds too simple, but you are your own master and have freedom of choice. Spend a lot of time with people who raise your spirits and make you feel good! You and your health will greatly benefit from it.

Source

Us: We are the absolute greatest influence on ourselves and our energy field! All of the preceding examples dim against the greatest source of positive or negative energy that lies within our own minds. Whether you think you are a positive or a negative person—you are right!

The stress that you experience is not someone else's fault; they may be the trigger, but you alone are the boss of your stress. Many people tighten up and become negative when outer influences, other people, or any of the preceding examples "stress them out." However, most people don't realize that it is purely their own reaction to those outer influences that causes the stress. Irritability, tight muscles, high blood pressure, fast heartbeat, and most illnesses are directly or indirectly caused by stress. According to my teacher, Mr. Domancic, almost all of illnesses today are caused by stress. It is all preventable through awareness coupled with a little positive attitude. How do you recognize stress?

> When my daughter Kylie asked me about stress, I didn't know what to say. How do you explain that to an eight-year-old? Plus, there was a six-year-old listening nearby.

"Well honey, it is like tension, or sadness, or negative thinking . . ."

"Daddy, what is negative thinking?"

Oh, boy . . . "OK, honey, let's try it this way: Imagine two guys staring out the window. It is pouring rain. One of them goes: "Grrrr! I hate this weather! I can't go out . . . I can't play golf . . . I can't do anything . . . I hate it!" And with that he stays angry, negative, and stressed all day. The other guy looks out and says: "Wow, look at that beautiful rain! It is so nice . . . so good for the grass and the plants . . . I can finally pick up my favorite book and just relax." He will stay happy, relaxed, and positive for the rest of the day. So we have two guys in the same situation: one all negative while the other is all positive, right?"

"Right," she said.

"Now comes the big question: Did either one of them change the weather? Of course not! This means that all the negative or positive happens only in our own minds. It is really up to us what we make out of a situation." That was the best I could do.

Only a week after our conversation, we drove to the Skatium, which is about an hour from our home, to go ice skating. When we arrived, we discovered that there was a hockey game on, and the Skatium was closed to public skating. Now what? I could just see my younger daughter's little lips turning down . . .

Suddenly, I heard Kylie: "Now, now, Karlyn," she said, "remember the two guys and the rain? Think positive!" she added.

All of a sudden, our troubles ended. We got some hot chocolate and we ended up watching a hockey game—their first hockey game ever. So what is stress? We are still not sure. Whatever it is, I know one thing: it is curable with hot chocolate!

Of course, hot chocolate may not be readily available, so you have to dig deep to prevent yourself from becoming self-destructive. If you have ever read *The Secret* or any other book that teaches how your thoughts become reality, then you know that it applies not only to the good and fuzzy thoughts but to the negative ones as well. Whatever you truly believe is exactly what eventually happens. I choose to think positive all the time and always see the glass as half full. It has worked well for me for more than twenty years. It may work for you, too!

Solution

To follow a positive thinking–based lifestyle, you have to change your core thinking. It is not enough to just "think positive"; it has to go deeper than that. For starters, you may have to change your vocabulary. Every word and thought carries positive or negative vibrations with it. Just thinking a word will change your energy field in that instant.

If you have never seen Masaru Emoto's pictures, you definitely should. Mr. Emoto took photographs of frozen water crystals under the microscope, comparing the beauty of mountain spring water crystals with those of dead Tokyo tap water. One day he realized that "adding emotions" to the water changed the crystals altogether. First, he asked some Buddhist monks to chant over the water, which resulted in beautiful frozen crystals. Later he realized that simply saying or even thinking a simple word would provide the same results. Finally, he learned that just writing down a single word on a piece of paper and placing it next to the water would do exactly the same. A negative word such as *hate* would result in a plain, dark, and ugly crystal. On the other hand, a positive word such as *love* would present itself as a brilliant crystal. Choose your thoughts, your words, and your writing wisely!

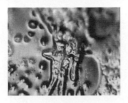

Hate (courtesy of
Masaru Emoto)

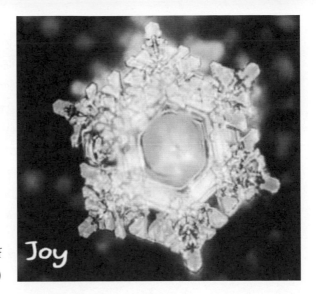

Joy (courtesy of
Masaru Emoto)

At one of my seminars a woman stood up and said: "Positive thinking doesn't really work. When I had a headache last time, I tried thinking positive but my headache remained!"

"What were you thinking?" I asked.

"No headache, no headache, no headache . . . but nothing happened." She said.

Of course not! In this case there was no positive thinking at all. "No" is a negative word. Repeating the word "headache" just reinforced the same. Instead, you should be thinking: "With every breath I take, I feel better and better." Or: "I feel more relaxed and happy with every passing moment." Or: "My neck muscles are relaxing and becoming mellow and soft. My head feels better every minute . . ."

Positive thinking requires a revamped dictionary. All the negative words should leave not only your vocabulary, but your thoughts as well. It is very challenging at the start, but soon you will find yourself thinking along those lines effortlessly.

This new dictionary is quite necessary since many negative things are so embedded in your subconscious that you can't ever change them. That is OK though. You do need a bit of negativity. The "fight-or-flight" reaction of your body cannot kick in without it. A good cry is very necessary sometimes as well. The first angry reaction after someone cuts you off on the highway may also be indispensable not only as your survivor instinct, but also as proof that you are human. However, all those reactions should last only a few seconds or maybe minutes, and then you have to let them go. Continuing to carry those thoughts may affect your energy field in the long run. Feel the anger for a moment, let it out, and let it go. Life goes on, and you only live in the moment. The driver may have cut you off in the past, but you don't really have a problem with him this very moment, do you?

It is preferred that you read up on some Zen philosophy or at least some books by Eckhart Tolle, which teach living in the now. In summary: many people shut out the very moment they are in because they concentrate too much on past problems—it consumes their lives and becomes a problem in the present. The missed opportunities, the mistakes, the past relationships, failed business deals, and such create stress and negative energy for you today when in fact you could have a wonderful, relaxing, and happy day instead. Thinking about the future is fine; however, when you get consumed by it, especially constantly delaying certain things (I will quit drinking, smoking, etc. in the future) or daydreaming about some goals that you don't really work on, these thoughts can also take away from the very moment you are in. You only live now! You may have noticed that when you do a certain activity that you love and that requires more concentration, you are truly happy. For some people, it is playing games or sports that puts them into the moment while, for others, it may be cooking or being with a loved one that will do the trick. Rock climbers or aerial artists have to fully concentrate on what they do since they could die any moment. They are in the Now, for sure!

I noticed that, when I ride my motorcycle on sharp mountain curves, I can't think of anything else, because it requires my full concentration since my life is in constant danger. Not only does it keep me in the moment, but it also keeps me happy, with a giant smile on my face!

If you feel you are drifting into negative territory outside this very moment, either take a deep breath and concentrate on it, or look at your hands and bring yourself back into this world and into this time. The funny thing is that you never really have a problem at this very moment!

My basic philosophy has helped me throughout the years—it may help you as well:

1. *Everything happens for a reason.* Whether you bring in higher powers, your life's lessons from the other side, or any other philosophical thinking, even logic would later show that this is true. If you don't see the reasons when certain things happen (they may be negative at that moment), don't worry; you will eventually discover them. Be content, and continue with your life.

2. *There is something positive in everything that happens!* It is enough to think about the t'ai chi symbol (yin and yang) or the basic atomic structure to know that everything is comprised of positive and negative aspects. If something negative happens, there surely is something positive attached to it. You may not see it at that moment, but you have to know that it is there. Not only believe it, but know it! *Many years ago, when I was lying in the hospital in Lake Havasu City with a shattered femur, I was thinking: "OK, what is positive here?" Then, a millisecond later, the positive thoughts started pouring in, and they still haven't stopped (for example, it is positive at this moment that I can write about this experience, and you will learn something new!):*

"I am in an awesome hospital; they put my leg back together; it is a nice room with a nice view; I am lucky my wife and my friends are nearby . . ." I was told that I wouldn't walk for six months. Instead, I used all my knowledge and was back teaching t'ai chi a month and a half later! *How positive is that?!* I am still able to bring it up after seventeen years. Even when someone dies, eventually, there will be something positive coming out of it. I know I would rather have my father back than the positive experiences that came since his death, but dying is part of life, and we can't avoid it. Again, there is something positive in everything, and whether you look for it or not, it is coming your way.

3. *Go with the flow.* Or, as the old Hungarian proverb says, *Don't piss against the wind!* Some things are not meant to be when we want them. We may not always know the reason for the things that happen around us (refer to philosophy #1). Nevertheless, timing is a good excuse, as are the circumstances. When the student is ready, the teacher will show up, says the Chinese proverb. Relax, and be happy!

5.
Becoming a Healer

We all had some unusual and unexplained experiences in our lives. I had too many to list. With time and education, these phenomena were eventually explained. However, one thing remained a mystery for many years of my young life—this "feeling" that I sometimes had in my hands, sometimes in my head. It would differ depending on whether I was alone or with other people. Not only did I feel things, but sometimes I would hear strange sounds or voices when no one was around.

I chose engineering for my future profession as I really had a knack for science, machines, and logic in general. I tried to suppress the other feelings since there was no reasonable explanation for them.

My first experience with feeling the energy between my hands came in my parents' living room, with the help of my dad's good friend who was a bit ahead of his time in the energy sciences. Once he showed me how to feel the energy and how to affect the energy field, all my engineering ambitions were pushed to the background. I quickly showed off my knowledge to my friends who teased me quite a bit at the beginning, but after a few pains were stopped, the mockery stopped as well. An ultramarathon-runner friend of mine had a life-long pain in his ankle that vanished after only a few minutes of my treatment. Another friend's migraine stopped after the first treatment. My great-grandmother was given only six months to live due to breast cancer that had spread throughout her body. She was eighty-five when I started practicing on her every chance I had. She lived another five years with nary a problem. She was old-fashioned and called the energy treatment "praying." "Are you praying over me?" she would ask each time. Whatever she called it, it worked!

However, I still wasn't convinced that this was my future. I was still looking for signs. I needed some validation.

One day my mom was complaining of a backache. By then, I was pretty confident that I could stop her pain. I asked her to step into the middle of the living room. We pretended that it was my office. It was a quiet fall afternoon with gray skies outside and nobody around. I stood behind her and ran my hand up and down her spine. I did that without touching her to feel the imbalance in her energy field. Once I found it, I proceeded to take off the excess energy, which is usually the source of pain. I virtually pulled the energy out of her field.

I will never forget *what happened next:*

All of a sudden, my mom started moving back! Her feet were still in the same spot, but her body leaned back, following my hand. When I moved my hand forward, her body moved forward. When I moved my hand back, she moved back!

I said: "Mom, what are you doing?"

"Nothing! What are you doing?" she shot back.

"I don't know. What are you doing?"

Our befuddled exchange went back and forth, synchronized with my mom's movement. We pretty much freaked out. Apparently, I was able to move her without touching her. It was frightening and exciting at the same time. Her pain did go away, but by then it wasn't the focus of the moment. I had this new power that I had to explore. The same evening when I went out with my friends, I told them what happened. Naturally, nobody believed me, so I had to try it on all of them. It worked! They weren't dropping like flies, but most of them moved. By the end of the night we were making bets for beer!

Not that I had too much of it, but I could just hear the voice deep in my mind: "Dude, do you need any more signs?!"

Sure enough, although I did finish my engineering degree, I ended up in the healing business after all. Twenty-plus years into it, I still follow the signs!

One of those signs came in the form of a TV report about Zdenko Domancic, a Croatian healer who by then puzzled most of Europe with his healing abilities. The small Adriatic island where he lived was inundated with people seeking healing. Aerial photos were showing hundreds of people snaking through the narrow streets of the island patiently waiting for their turn. Many of them were holding their sick children, while others were pushing their loved ones in wheelchairs. It was amazing to see and to hear the reports of miraculous healings performed by this man. The part that was most exciting for me came in the form of psychokinesis—Mr. Domancic was moving and even bending people without touching them, sometimes from several feel away. Finally, I found someone I could learn from.

My meeting with Domancic came much later with the help of a professor from a Belgrade college who measured my energy and highly recommended that I change professions and become a full-time healer (all of these encounters are detailed in my first book: *Biotherapy: A Healing for the 21st Century*). Needless to say, I heeded his advice. I became an established healer (or biotherapist) in my former country before moving to the United States.

I had lost touch with Domancic during the Balkan Wars and had no idea where he could be. One night, some sixteen years after we last saw each other, I had a strange dream about us wrapping up a seminar together. "It was great to see you, but it would be nicer if we met in person again." he said. I woke up with a strange feeling but gave it no more thought.

All of this happened several months after a weeklong seminar that I taught in Denmark. At that time, I was already teaching not only in the United States but internationally as well. I was contacted by a documentary crew that was filming Domancic, asking me for an interview. They found me through the Danish website, which praised the seminar. They were already finishing their project and wanted to contact some of Domancic's former students, inevitably connecting us after so many years. We do have to listen to our dreams and the messages they convey!

Domancic remains very well known and very active in Slovenia. The documentary, *Think About It* (2006), has some amazing

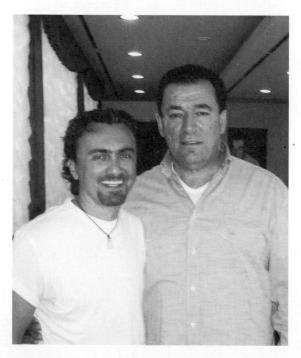

Author with Zdenko Domancic in 2006

footage and some detailed studies on Domancic and a few of his patients. The filmmakers claim that he had healed more than a million people!

The good news is that, after a million patients, one figures out what works and what doesn't. We can now reap the benefits of that experience. Thank you, Domancic!

After living in the United States for a while, I started teaching t'ai chi for larger groups. Naturally, I not only explained the body's movements, but also talked about the energy flow. This progressed to showing my students how to feel and how to see the energy. To my surprise, they did really well. That is when I realized that anyone can do what I do—at least to a certain degree.

You don't have to be mystical or extraordinary to step into the world of energy healing. Truly, anyone can become a healer. As I said, we were all born with a special talent. If healing is not your talent, it doesn't prevent you from doing it by any means. You may not be suited to do it as a profession, but you can certainly heal friends and family or anyone else who needs help. All you need is a clear mind, determination, and desire—the same substances you need to learn anything else.

6.

Feel the Energy

Most people have felt the energy hundreds or even thousands of times in their lifetime, without ever knowing it. Many times we don't pay attention to certain things until someone points them out to us. Such is the case with the energy. Think of the experience of hugging, or stopping your child's pain, or the movie theatre, or the telephone call . . .

Feeling the energy is relatively easy, and once you have learned how to do it, you will never forget it—just like riding a bicycle! About 80 percent of people will be able to do it upon their first attempt and another 10 percent at their second. For some reason, there are a small number of individuals who can't feel the energy, but they may be able to see it. It is altogether possible to heal without feeling or seeing it though.

Once learned, the feeling intensifies with practice. The more you practice, the more refined your senses will become. Eventually, you will feel someone's energy and the imbalances in it within seconds.

Let's begin . . .

First exercise

For your first exercise, lift your arms up straight in front of you with your palms facing down. Let your hands drop with your fingers relaxed all the way. Now lift your fingers up, so your hands are perfectly aligned with your outstretched arms. Repeat two or three times until you can differentiate the amount and location of muscular tension between the two positions. There should be just a bit of tension in the upper part of your hands as well as in your fingers when they are up. This tension will provide a guideline to the feeling that accompanies the radiation of energy from your hands.

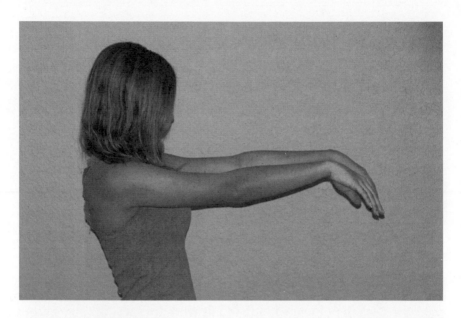

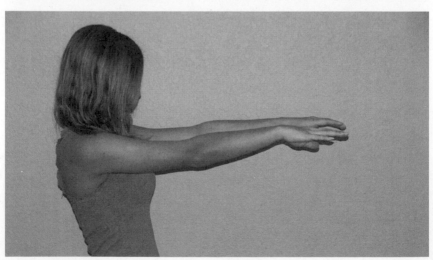

Now, still maintaining the light tension in your hands, let your elbows drop, and visualize holding a basketball between your perfectly parallel hands. The better you visualize it, the faster you will feel it. Once you think you have it, give it a little squeeze: let your palms come together by an inch and then pull them back to the starting position. Repeat several times. What do you feel? Can you feel the ball? Can you feel the resistance between your hands—as if you were pressing an actual ball or balloon? Have you ever played with magnets—when you try to push them together and they resist? That is how this feels. Magnets attract each other as long as the positive side faces the negative side of the other magnet. However, when you try to push the same polarities together, they resist with

varying degrees relative to their size. Your hands act like weak magnets. You won't need major muscle power to push your hands together, but if you are able to feel the energy, there will be a slight resistance that is quite amazing the first time (and every time!) you feel it.

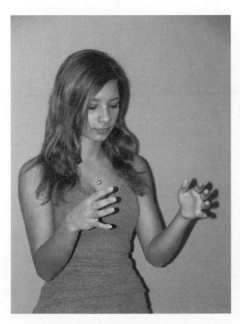
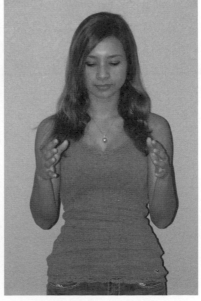

Continue bouncing your hands back and forth a little faster. Some of you will feel the ball much better this way. Now, start getting your hands closer and closer to each other with every bounce. You may feel a subtle difference at certain points. You have several layers of energy around you, and some of you may be able to feel them. Don't worry if you don't.

What else do you feel? Can you feel the warmth between your hands? Isn't it strange that you can actually feel it—since your hands are both the same temperature? Also, can you feel tingling? It won't feel like pins and needles—but tingling nevertheless.

Now bring your hands to an inch distance from each other, and hold them there for a minute. Make sure that your hands are flat and your fingers are straight. Can you still feel the previous sensations? Some of them intensified, didn't they? At this point, if you move your fingers just a little bit, especially if you bend them a tiny bit and then straighten them back up several times, you may feel as if your knuckles need lubrication. They feel a bit squeaky, don't they? All of what you are feeling at this point is the sensation that accompanies the radiation of bioenergy.

After holding your hands at an inch distance for a while, start circling them. Do you remember the feeling when trying to push the magnets together? They wouldn't go of course, but they would try to avoid each other in a circular fashion. That is the exact feeling you may experience here. Your hands will follow a certain circular path. This is a bit harder to feel than the previous exercise, but if your arms are relaxed enough and your hands are just a bit tight, you will feel the gentle circle and the subtle resistance. Keep trying! Once you feel it, you may increase the size of the circle and experiment to see how far you can separate your hands while still feeling the energy. You will be surprised by the size of the energy ball!

Now bring your hands back together, and stop at an inch distance. After about five seconds, slowly pull your hands apart. Can you feel the resistance to this motion? This resistance shows you that the "magnets" are not only between your hands, but also on the outside of them. As a matter of fact, they are everywhere since the energy surrounds your entire being. We use our hands for this exercise because they have the most sensory receptors. Thus, we will use our hands for not only our everyday tasks, but for healing as well. We can heal with any part of our body indeed, but the hands are the most effective "feelers."

If you have trouble feeling the energy, you can try a little trick: press down hard on the middle of the palm of your hand with the other hand's thumb for a few seconds. Repeat on the other palm. This pressure will increase the sensation in those spots, so you can feel the energy easier. Later on, with some practice, you may not need this trick at all. Repeat the previous exercises with this newfound sensation.

These drills are designed to give you the best sensitivity for bioenergy. Practice them until you reach a point where you can feel the energy within seconds of trying.

Second exercise

Start the next exercise by repeating what we have just done. Once you feel the energy between your hands, turn your palms up and bring them close to your face. Now, without touching, move your hands in a circular motion as if you were washing your face. Keep your hands a few inches away, and cover most of your face with every pass. Can you feel the heat radiating from your hands? Can you feel the heat radiating from your face? You may also experience a bit of pressure in your sinuses, especially if you ever had any sinus issues. If you go around your ears, you may sense some pressure there as well. Continue moving your hands in a path that covers your entire head and pull your hands down on the side, just above your shoulders.

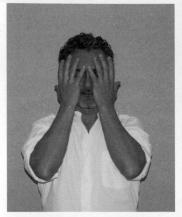
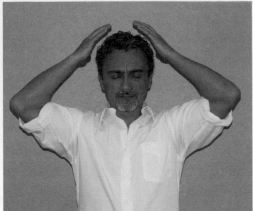
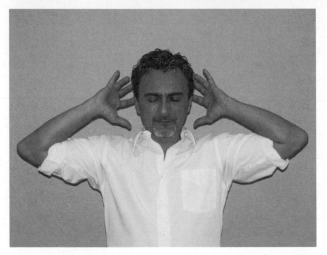

If you ever have a headache, you can reduce or stop it with the same movements, with the addition of coming down the sides of your head with your hands, all the way to an extended arm a bit away from your body. You should end this move by shaking your hands to dissipate the excess energy. This energy literally sticks to your hands, and if not shaken off, it will remain and may even cause pain or discomfort there. Incidentally, stopping your own pain is the hardest thing to do. It is much easier to stop other people's pain than your own. A difference in polarity and the levels of energy (or charge) help the process between two individuals. Either way, do shake your hands to free them of the excess energy.

At the very beginning of my career, before anyone explained the process to me, I used to stop someone's pain, and I would end up with painful hands or even headaches. I didn't know that the energy would stick to my hands and stay there if I failed to shake it off. I would like to spare you that experience. Holding your hands under running water for a minute or so works as well, but the shaking of hands is more effective and instantaneous.

Let's pause here for visualization purposes. Since it may still be hard to grasp the concept of energy—never mind the actual feeling—we can use other mental pictures to clarify things, especially shaking off the energy.

Think of your aura as if it were jello. If you had a bowl of it and wanted to empty it with your bare hands, could you do it in one move without turning over the bowl? Probably not. You could grasp some of it with your hands, while some would just stick to them automatically. You'd pull your hands out and shake the jello off. Then you would repeat the process until the bowl was empty. If you can visualize working with jello around the body, then you can understand how the energy sticks to your hands and why you have to make several passes. It is quite simple to understand this way, isn't it?

Third exercise

Begin the next exercise by holding the ball again. Once you feel it, start moving your right hand up your left inner forearm. Once you reach the inner elbow, move back to your hand with the same slow speed, and repeat several times. Can you feel the heat in your hand and/or forearm?

Once you feel it, move to the outside of your forearm. It is a bit harder here since your skin is thicker and less sensitive.

The same exercise can be repeated with only the forefinger moving up and down. Once you feel with your finger (and once you feel the

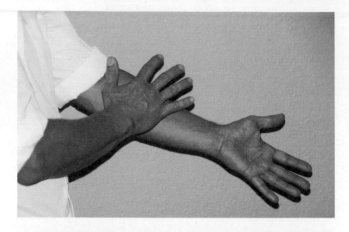

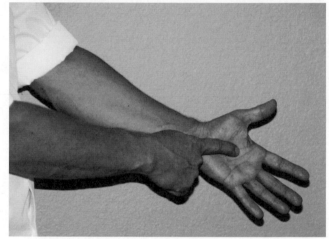

finger with your forearm), move it down to your hand, and circle it around the middle of your palm. Can you feel it? It almost tickles, doesn't it? These finger exercises have no major therapeutic purpose but are fun and help to raise your energy awareness.

Fourth exercise

Start the next exercise as usual: feeling the ball first. Next, bring the ball down to your stomach area, and separate your hands. Keep either hand in front of the stomach for about ten to fifteen seconds, and then start circling it clockwise. Continue until you can feel it clearly. This motion, when performed on others, would have beneficial effects for the digestive system, especially the large intestines. It helps very much with constipation (it takes about fifty circles with the speed of one to two seconds per pass). The opposite move (counterclockwise) is a remedy for diarrhea. You can perform this with both hands interlocked for added effect.

> *Several years ago, I spent fifteen days with a group in Egypt, and this was a lifesaver. Many didn't heed the warning not to drink the water. I had to perform it on at least a third of the group. They were very thankful!*

At this time, you have enough feeling in your hands to start exploring your own body first and then others'. Feel your own shoulders, elbows, knees, and so on. Once you sense the differences in all these areas, get a partner, and explore their energy.

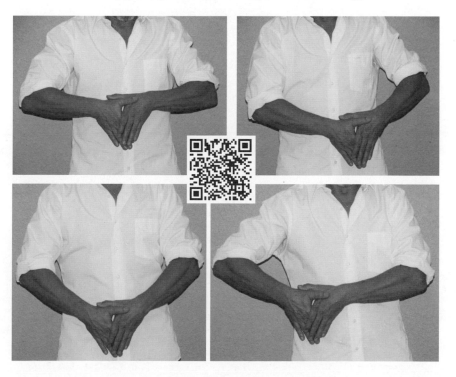

7.

Scan the Body

For this exercise, you obviously need a partner. Anyone will do; however, if you want to take your energy diagnostic abilities a step farther, find someone who is not closely related to you. It doesn't have to be somebody off the street, just a person not in your immediate family or group of friends. This will let you explore their energy without any predetermined knowledge, prejudice, or wishful thinking regarding the person. Also, there will be less of a possibility for your energies to be on the same level. Practice on someone you can be totally neutral with.

Supposedly, the great scientist, Nikola Tesla never shook hands with anyone, believing that such an act would equalize their energies for many hours and would hurt his genius.

Crossing hands

Start and finish each healing session with these moves. Don't expect anything too fancy; your hands won't follow any strict routes or meridians, and they won't cross exactly over the chakras. Their purpose is simply to open (at the beginning) and close (at the end) the aura. In other words, it is the mark of the beginning of a treatment, where your energy gently enters the other person's aura. At the end of your session, the same moves will not only mark the conclusion, but will smooth out the surface of the aura to make sure it is even. In addition, these moves reconnect the left and right sides of the damaged mind/body link.

Stand in front of your partner, and put your leading hand above their head for a second or two. Now, as if you were an ambidextrous beauty queen in a parade, wave with both hands in a wide fashion (so that your hands crisscross) all the way down below the waistline to a point where you have to bend at your waist just a little bit. You will cross your hands approximately three to four times. The palms of your hands will face the body almost directly at the top while they will gently move to a 45 degree angle toward the middle and finally to almost horizontal at the bottom. There is a very light tension in the fingers; otherwise, the whole move is quite relaxed. Repeat the same motions while standing behind your partner. You may do a couple of passes on each side if you wish—no harm done. It is the exact same procedure at the end of the treatment.

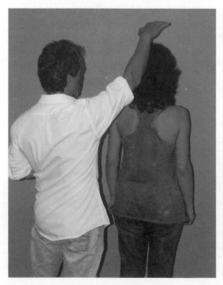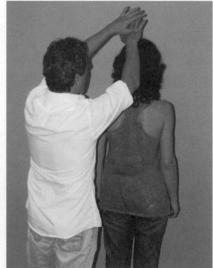

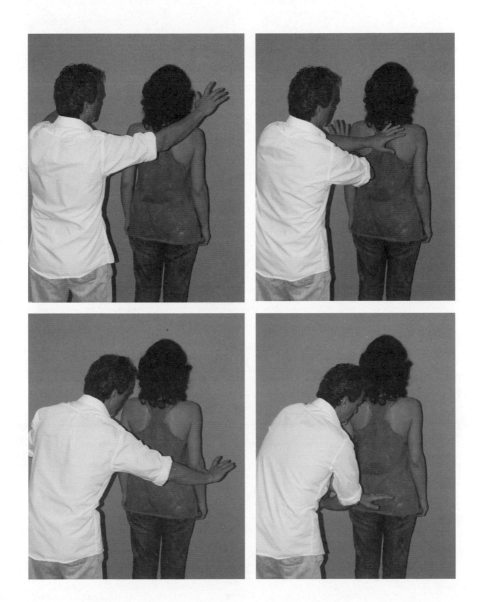

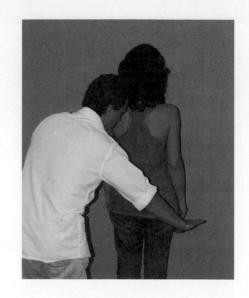

Examining the aura

While you are standing behind your partner, lift your hand (the one that is more sensitive, if either one is) above his or her head, and slowly move it down toward the bottom of the spine and below. Keep your hand about 4–5 inches distance from the body. Make sure that the palm of the hand is facing your partner. Repeat the movement up and down the spine several times at a comfortable speed that lets you feel the energy the best. Can you feel slight differences in the field? They may come as warmth, cold, tingling, pressure, suction, or a certain magnetic push or pull. All of those deviations from the regular "ball" feeling are clues to imbalances in the field. It would be a good idea later on to find someone with pre-established problems (neck pain, lower back pain, asthma, etc.) on which to practice to aid in validating your sensitivity. With most adults, there is a good chance that you will feel differences around the neck and lower back areas since those are the most vulnerable to stress in our modern times. Repeat all your movements several times, and stop wherever you feel these differences. For now, cover only the spine and the back of the head. Those areas—the central nervous system—have the strongest energy and are the easiest to feel.

Once you have found all the problem areas of the spine, you may move on to the rest of the back. Again, work your way down from the top of your partner's head, this time covering the whole back in a slow, side to side, sweeping motion. Pay attention to all the signals that you receive; validate them first by rechecking them and then by asking for feedback from your partner. You are still in the learning process, so don't expect to feel everything perfectly or clearly. These are all exercises that will sharpen your senses and add to your skills.

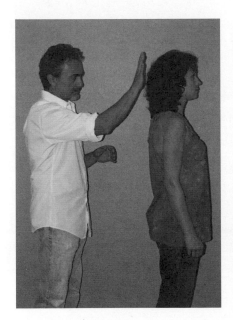 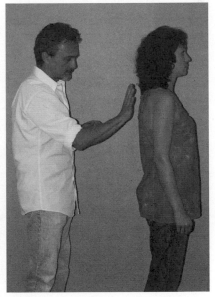

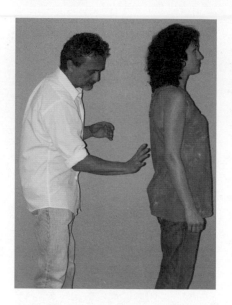
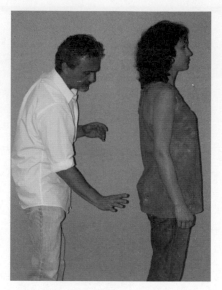

When you finish examining the back, move to the front, and start the same process from the top of the head and down. Feel the forehead, the sinuses, neck, chest, stomach, liver/gallbladder, spleen, intestines, reproductive organs, while still keeping the established distance of around 4–5 inches from the body. What do you feel? Where are the areas of imbalances? Again, validate what you feel, and then ask for feedback.

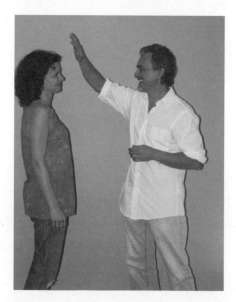

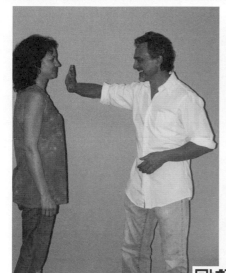

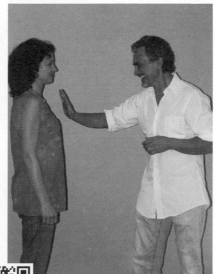

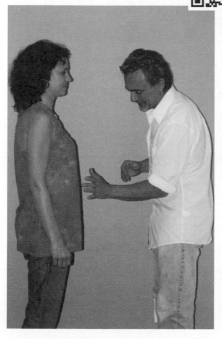

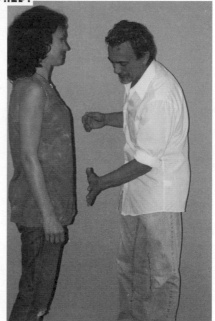

When you master the feeling of the energy around the body, you may step away from it and try to feel the edge of the energy field which we know is roughly as far as one can reach. You may feel the exact magnetic repulsion sensation you have felt with the ball. See if you can feel the density and smoothness around the entire field. It is quite an amazing experience, isn't it?

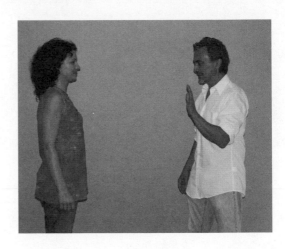

The entire scanning process should be repeated once you are done with the healing session. This will give you a validation of what you have completed or healed, and will also give you a clue to which areas are the most problematic. At the next session, this same procedure will show you even better where more help and work may be needed. Some weak imbalances that you have felt the first time may be completely gone. That is a clue that those were nothing serious. Sometimes you will pick up on totally insignificant imbalances, such as at the stomach immediately after a heavy meal. The next time there may be no signals at all.

Before we move on to the actual healing, you may want to learn how to . . .

8.

See the Energy

As mentioned before, it is not necessary to feel or to see the energy in order to perform any healing. However, since most people can learn to see the energy within a few minutes, why not try it?! Personally, I don't use this ability when I work one-on-one with my clients although I may take a quick glance at them when I see them the first time. However, this is one of those abilities that help the visualization process when performing long-distance healing (LDH). It is also quite cool to see the auras at some special events or occasions, such as looking at the singers' energy at the opera or the actors' energy at the theatre. When they are at their very best, you can literally see a bubble coming out of the top of their heads!

For the first exercise, choose a calm and plain background. It is best if it is a one-color wall indoors, with lighting that is not too bright. Some people prefer white while others like darker colors. You will find your favorite as well. Facing the bare wall, lift your straight arms, with the elbows slightly bent, to eye level. The palms of the hands should face you, fingers spread, with the fingertips pointing at each other. Leave about 4" of distance between them. You will need some concentration at this point: focus your eyes at the area between the fingertips of the middle fingers (sure, you can choose any other two fingers, but these are the longest and thus the most convenient ones to look at). Don't look at the fingers and don't look at the background. Your focus should be entirely on the area between the fingertips of the middle fingers. What do you see? Can you see the connection between the fingertips? At first, it will be very faint, but the more you focus on the exact distance and the area between the fingertips, without glancing to the wall or the fingers themselves, the clearer it will become. Is it a bit hazy, watery, foggy, misty, or smoky? Does it resemble the air above hot asphalt in the summertime? Whichever it reminds you of the most, it doesn't matter. Either way, you are seeing it! About 90 percent of people can see this in their first try. If you don't see anything, you have to adjust your focus or change the background or the lighting.

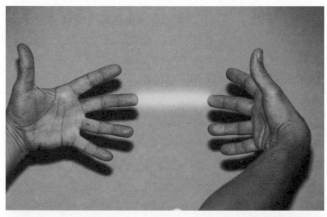

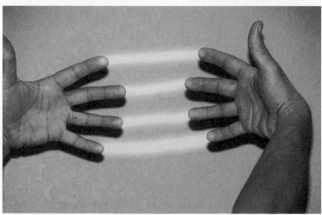

Once you can see the connection between the two fingers, you may try to see it between all of them. All it takes is adjusting your focus so you have all the fingers in your sight. What happens when you move one hand up and down an inch or two? Can you see the connections moving as well?

Now keep the left hand up as before with the fingers spread and only the forefinger of the right hand pointing at the forefinger of the left. First establish the same vision as before: see the connection between the two forefingers. Now move the right forefinger slowly down. You'll see how it connects first to the left middle finger, then the ring finger, and finally the pinky. If the distance is far enough, it will keep the connection with all the fingers!

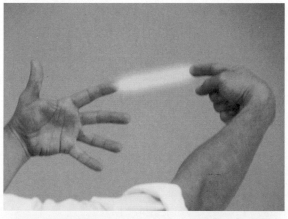

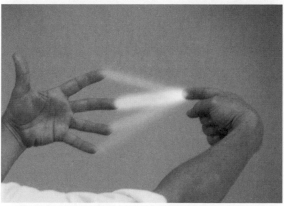

Look at the right forefinger by itself. Keep it at arm's length, eye level and pointing up. You have to adjust your sight to look at the area around the forefinger, without concentrating on the background (which is still a plain wall). Your focus is not on the finger, but around it. Can you see the haziness around the finger? If you move your focal point to be the top of the finger, right above the fingertip, the density will be a bit different. Can you see it? It is a little bit thicker and brighter, almost resembling a funnel. This little tornado shape comes from the energy center of the fingertip, which is also known as a chakra.

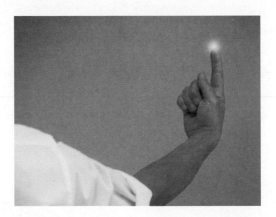

The crown chakra

The term *chakra* comes from India, and it refers to the energy centers of the body. There are seven major chakras around the midline of the body and twenty-one secondary chakras elsewhere. Additionally, each fingertip and toe-tip is a mini chakra. Some other theories count nine or even eleven major chakras. We won't get into a discussion about these—let the scientists decide. It is not necessary to know the exact location or number of chakras in order to perform healing. It is a nice exercise to try to see them though, so let's see the crown chakra for our next exercise.

Have a friend stand against the same plain wall you have been using. Stand about ten feet or more in front of him/her. Look at the area right above his/her head. In a similar fashion as looking at the fingertip, try not to look at the wall or at your friend. Your focus should be on the area (and distance) right above the head. Can you see the same haziness as you saw above your finger? It is obviously bigger and brighter. You may see the funnel shape easier as well. It may appear to be like a shadow, so to remove all doubt, try the next simple exercise.

Tell your friend to visualize the happiest moment of his/her life, and watch what happens. The aura above their head starts to rise! It may not appear all straight or perfect. It may even pull to one side. However, it will be super bright and happy. As mentioned before, try this exercise at the theatre or the opera. You will be blown away by the size of the energy bubble above the singers' or actors' heads!

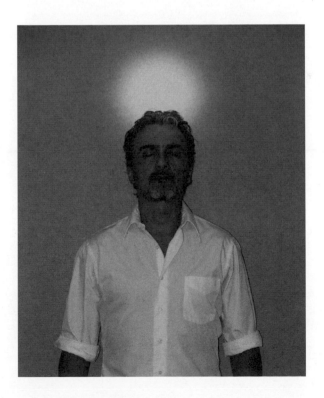

If you want to see more drastic changes, tell your friend to think of the saddest moment of his or her life. The aura may darken and shrivel up to almost nothing.

The preceding exercises are even more fun when practiced in a group. It is nice to know that everyone else sees the same, and you are not imagining things.

You can practice seeing the energy around just about anyone. You will also see big differences at various locations from restaurants, schools, court rooms, theatre, to public transportation, airports, and so on.

Some of you may develop a keen eye for the aura and may choose to rely on your vision to perform the energy diagnoses, but most people are quite happy with just feeling the energy.

9.
Bioenergy Healing

The universe is governed by some simple rules: gravity pulls, water flows, wind blows, the earth spins, and so on. Similarly, we have a certain system of movements to regulate bioenergy. These laws are very easy to learn and implement.

As far as our bodies are concerned, there is really no "bad" energy, just too much or too little of it. Most of the time healing is all about taking energy away or adding energy in order to restore the balance in the field. Thus, you have to learn how to perform those tasks.

When there is too much energy, it is associated with pain, inflammation, hyperactivity, and such.

Too little energy means less protection and weaker shield (frail immune system), which is associated with most illnesses.

There is also the possibility of a separate energy field within a field, such as in case of cancer and tumors.

Basic hand moves and positions

The most basic hands-on-healing is exactly that: hands-on. That was the first form of healing dating back to the dawn of mankind. It is part of our instinct: when we get hurt, we immediately put our hand on the painful spot. When our child gets hurt, we put our hand on their painful area as well. Sometimes we rub it or kiss it, but the hand is always involved and is always touching.

When performing healing at a very basic stage, where we don't even know whether we should give energy or take it away, it is enough to tighten up our hand just a little bit (remember?) and put it on the area to be healed. You and your subject will probably feel the warmth, tingling, and pressure. Your bodies (as well as higher selves) will know what to do even if you don't. There will be an energy exchange between the two of you no matter what. The tighter hands will just make that happen easier and faster. If there is too little energy in the touched spot, your subject's body will pull the energy out of your hand. Contrarily, if there is too much energy, your subject's body will give it to your hands. In that case, you better get rid of it by shaking your hands off—like shaking the jello off your hands; otherwise, your hands may start hurting.

Next up would be holding the (slightly tightened) hand a few inches above the problem area. This not only allows you to actually feel the energy—instead of feeling the skin with your regular sensory receptors—but it also enhances the energy flow by a small percentage. This is due to involving extra layers of the energy field. The distance here should be around 2–6 inches, but it is really a personal preference. With experience, you will know exactly where your hand should be.

Circling the hand over the problem area at that distance would enhance the energy flow yet again since now we are affecting the area from different angles. We also have the advantage of feeling the energy from those angles, which sometimes gives us an indication to a better hand position for enhanced healing.

> As a general rule, we move the hands clockwise to add energy and counterclockwise to take it away.

There are other ways to enhance the energy flow to much higher levels. These maneuvers include concentrated energy flow from your solar plexus (the area right above your stomach), your third eye (the area between your eyebrows), or your brain. We will discuss some of them a bit later.

In general, there are only three major procedures that we can perform with the energy field: take energy, give energy, and balance (or spread) energy. All the other movements are just part of these three.

Taking energy

Dealing with too much energy is obvious: we have to take it away in order to find the balance. All pain, inflammation, and any type of hyper- anything is usually a sign of excess energy. Many times, relief comes within minutes of taking the surplus away or even during the procedure itself. The fast pain relief doesn't just work on headaches but on other pain as well, such as toothaches and earaches. Some pain that is more "physical" in nature may take longer or will be hard to stop altogether. Such is the case with broken bones, extremely pulled or torn muscles, and some other difficult muscle injuries. Just as the body sends pain signals to the brain when an injury happens, it also sends extra energy to protect the area—a process that increases the pain, too. In the case of a headache, it is easy to remove the extra energy when there is no physical attachment to it. However, with an actual physical injury, the body will keep sending the energy to continuously protect the area and speed up the healing process. This brings up a dilemma of whether you should attempt to stop pain when it may slow the recovery process. No worries—there is a fine line where the pain can be reduced while still helping the recovery. As long as there is energy moving, the natural processes are at work, such as in the case of the river versus the pond. The river flows; thus its water is always replenished and fresh while the pond's water is stagnant and stale. Which one is healthier? Having said that, you need to learn how to get that energy moving—in this case away from the body. The rules are very simple:

> To take away energy, always go from medial (middle) to lateral (side), and superior (top) to inferior (bottom).

With circular moves, always go counterclockwise. You may also pull the energy out at 90 degrees away from the body (pulling movements).

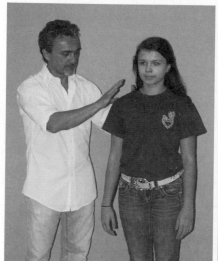
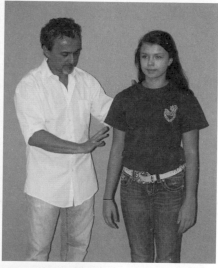

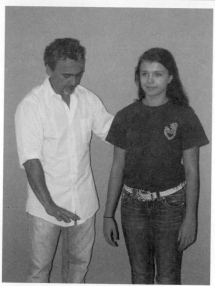

Take away energy: move from medial to lateral

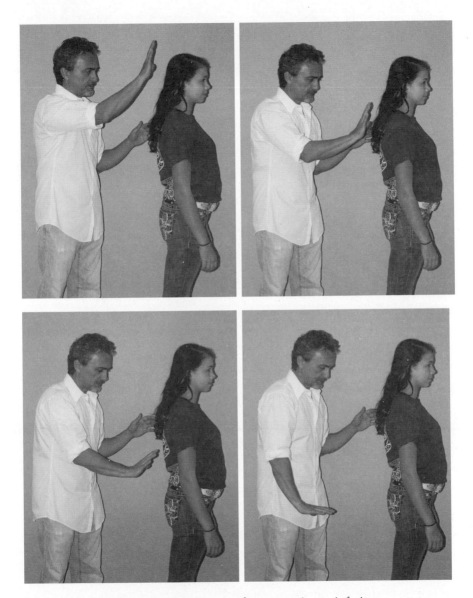

Take away energy: move from superior to inferior

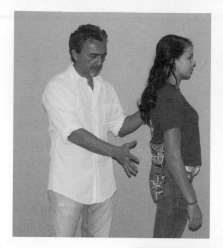
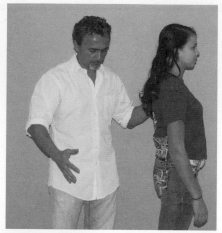

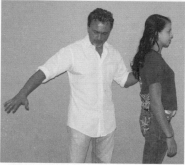

Take away energy: pull away from subject at 90 degree angle

As you learned before, hands-on itself will do the trick to a certain extent. When visualizing the jello, we tried to grab it and throw it away. Here, our goal is to learn to take the easy path. One variation is to pull the jello out at a straight angle and release or shake off the excess far away from the body (arm's length will do). If you want to grab more energy, you may circle the area a few times counterclockwise, like the cotton candy maker at the county fair, before pulling it out and throwing it away. Always shake your hands off a few times. Repeat until the pain is gone. All of these movements are done with your palm facing the body.

Sometimes the pain just doesn't want to stop. Other times, it is in an area where you simply can't pull it straight out. Yet other times, especially around the neck, lower back, and the spine in general, it is so concentrated that this method is just too sluggish. In all those cases, it is much easier to drag the energy down the spine or out toward the extremities and only then away from the body.

How do you know when you are done? The most certain way, of course, is when the pain stops. However, many times it won't stop right away, although there will be a significant reduction in pain. If your subject is comfortable enough with it, you may stop. There may be further pain reduction in the next minutes or hours as the body adjusts. If you have tried to reduce pain for more than fifteen minutes in one area and there is not an ounce of difference, it may be one of those rare occasions where you need to add energy to a painful area. This is very uncommon, but not impossible. For this purpose, I have developed a foolproof method that we will discuss in the next chapter.

Adding energy

Lack of energy is the cause (or consequence) of most health problems. In such cases, we need to add energy to restore the balance and thus help the body heal itself. The changes induced by the added energy take a bit longer to manifest than the sometimes immediate results of the pain relief treatments since the body needs more time to adjust and to hold on to the fresh energy. It is similar to starting a training routine. You can't just walk into a gym and bench press two hundred pounds on your first day. It takes time to condition your muscles. If you overdo it, your body will have to deal with the excess lactic acid and pain. Similarly, your body has to be conditioned to hold onto the extra energy you have added. There may even be a little discomfort, pain, or hyperactivity as a result of too much energy added—although these are rare occurrences that don't last long and may actually speed up the healing process (almost like the healing crises that some medicines and homeopathic remedies induce).

Aside from the hands-on method, there are many other ways to increase the body's energy:

> To give energy, always go from lateral to medial, and inferior to superior. With circular moves, always go clockwise. You may also push energy into the field at a 90 degree angle to the body.

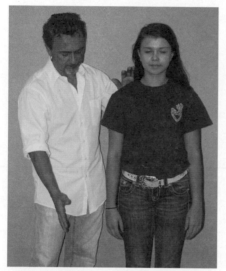
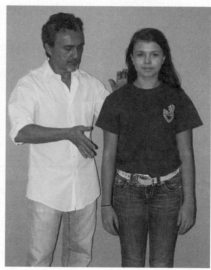

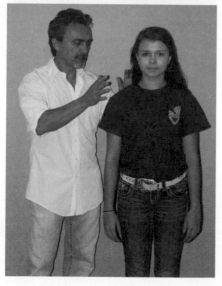

Add energy: move from lateral to medial, from inferior to superior (clockwise motion)

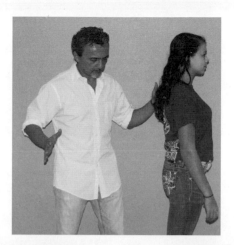

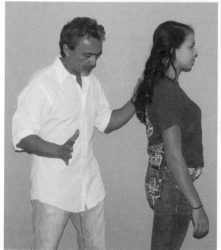
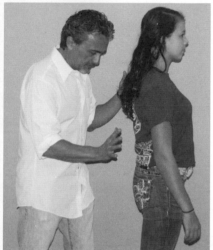

Add energy: push toward subject at 90-degree angle

Your hand will once again face the body as you add energy. This time you are rebuilding the jello sculpture. You may visualize smoothing it out as you add it, but it is not necessary. Your higher self will do most of the job.

How many times do we circle when adding energy? In general, it can go from a few circles up to about fifty. We will discuss this in the next chapter where the full treatments are explained.

How do you know when you are done? This is a bit harder than in the case of pain. With experience, you will actually feel the saturation of energy in the given field or even feel how your hands stop emitting the energy, just like when the green light turns on within your battery charger. There will be less tingling, and the tension will reduce in your hand. However, those feelings may be too subtle for you to notice at the beginning of your healing career. For that reason, in the next chapter you will learn the approximate amount of time you should spend on each case. The rest will come with experience.

Balancing the energy

These moves are also called the "crossing movements" and are used at the beginning and at the end of each treatment, regardless of whether you add or take energy. They serve several purposes:

1. At the beginning of the treatment, they let the energies of the therapist and subject "familiarize" with each other, as well as let the therapist open the subject's energy to "let himself in."
2. At the end of the treatment, these moves help seal or close the energy field by smoothing it out to prevent any areas from having too much energy, thus preventing pain or hyperactivity. It also marks the end of the treatment like the dot at the end of a sentence.
3. At localized areas, these moves help balance the energy for a gentle, even finish.
4. They reconnect the communication between the left and the right side of the body/brain.

As explained before (and this is worth repeating), facing our subject, we start above the top of the head by just holding one or both hands relaxed for a few seconds. This helps connect the two energy fields. With a gentle, circular path we move our hands down and cross them at several places in front of the body. As our hands

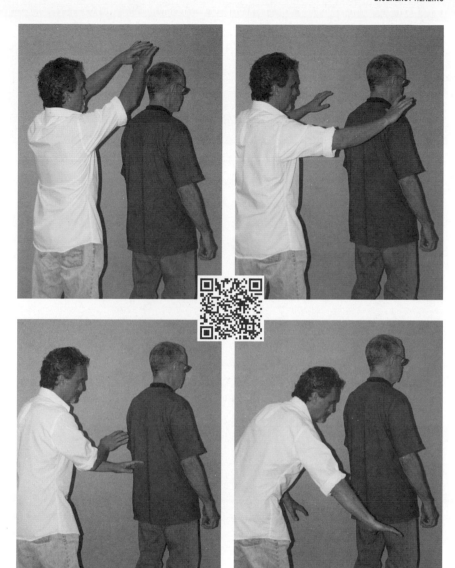

Balancing energy: crossing movements

move down, they will turn the palms naturally from facing the body to facing the floor. As they reach the lowest point (while we are still standing up), we move them up again in a smooth circular motion on the outside of the body (now without crossing) back to the top of the head. You may repeat once or twice if you wish. Do the same behind the back as well. All of this can be done with one hand if so desired.

For the localized areas, the approach is a little bit different. For instance, after working on the head, we can finish with a few crossing moves from above the head and down as if smoothing out a basketball. The hands should be slightly tight but not too much. Repeat five to seven times, and then move on to the rest of the body. At other places, you may just want to think of "smoothing the jello"—a few short waves to finish the specific area you have worked on.

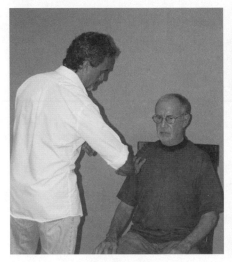
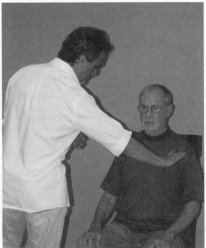

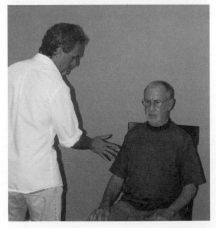

Cleansing movement

Additional movements

In the same category as balancing, we can include the "**Cleaning Movements**," which consist of moving the hand left and right a couple of times and then out of the aura followed by shaking off the hand a few times. This is also done with relaxed hands. Its purpose is to improve the function of select areas or organs. For instance, we always perform this above the heart following the treatment in that area, just to spread the energy a bit for a gentle finish.

Provoking the energy

This movement is designed to provoke, irritate, or awaken a certain area. It is a pure stimulation of the energy by tensing up the fingers and shaking or vibrating them as if playing the piano super fast. If done right, this sends a large amount of energy through our fingers into the problem area. Most people will feel this movement as a tingling sensation.

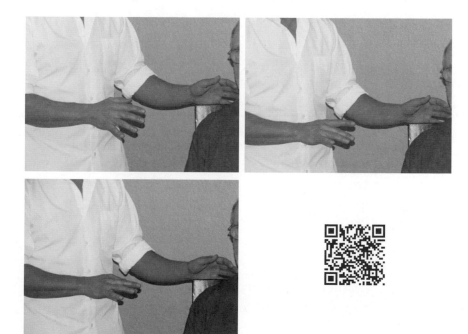

Ripping out the energy

This is a rare move that is used in treating tumors. We try to weaken the tumor's energy as we strengthen the rest of the body's energy.

With tight hands and fingers, we grasp the energy and literally rip it out of the body. As soon as our hands are far enough—about an arm's length from the body—we shake the hands off, and repeat five to seven times.

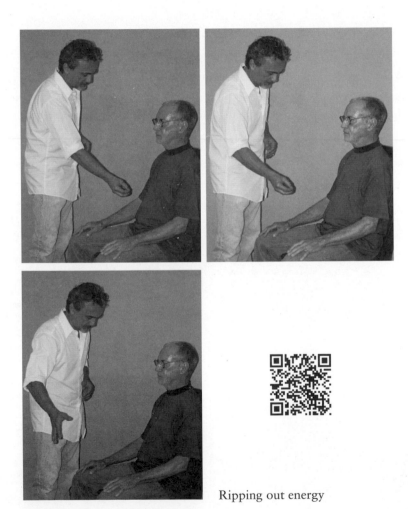

Ripping out energy

Waving (positive)

This move is also called positive therapy and, just like some of the previous procedures, was developed by Mr. Domancic many moons ago. It is one of his signature movements and is not found in any other energy balancing method. It is usually done toward the end of the treatment to not only load the energy, but also to jump-start the energy flow (the river) by pushing the energy up the front of the body. This is done with the subject sitting down with his/her feet on a chair, legs straight. We stand next to the legs and push the energy up the front of the body by tensing up the hands and fingers, moving them from below the feet to above the top of the head. All of this is done several inches from the body, so we will avoid accidentally hitting the person. Let the hands relax on the way down, and repeat rapidly with tense fingers on the way up. This ensures pushing the energy up, thus jump-starting the flow, as a plunger clears out pipes. It is also helpful to follow our hands with our eyes—all the way beyond the top of the head.

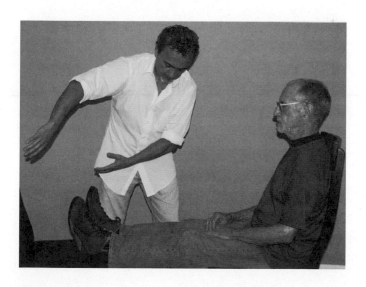

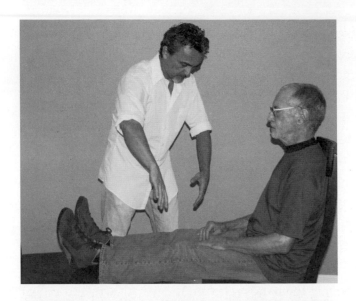

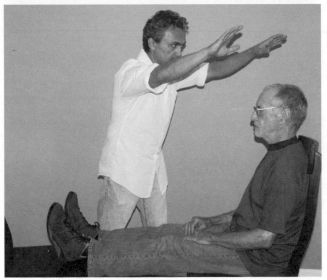

Waving
(positive)

Finishing moves: the tap

If you can imagine each cell in your body having its own internal clock, then you can imagine those clocks getting out of sync every time there is an energy imbalance in the system. Some of those clocks will run too fast while others may stay a bit behind, contributing to the overall chaos. When you get a biotherapy treatment, it is quite relaxing not only to your body, but to your entire energy field, including the clocks. At the end of the treatment, right after the final crossing movements behind the back, we can take advantage of that relaxed state by giving it a shock in the form of a quick yet not too powerful tap on the upper trapezius muscles. This creates a shock

to the relaxed system that instantaneously stops all the internal clocks for a split second. Once the shock is over, they all start working together in sync. This is not only a helpful surprise, but also a nice way to mark the end of the treatment.

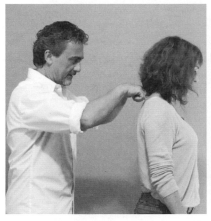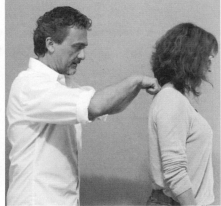

The tap

10.
The Procedure

Now that you know all the moves, it is just a matter of putting them together in the right order for you to become a serious healer. It is like a story: it has a beginning, a conflict, and a resolution. You start, you work, you finish.

The procedure:

- Crossing (opening) movements
- Assessment
- Treatment (adding energy, taking away energy, other treatments as needed)
- Reassessment (if needed)
- Waving (if needed)
- Reassessment (if needed)
- Crossing (closing) movements
- Finish/Tap

Crossing (opening) movements

We always start with the **crossing movement,** front and back. In some cases, it is enough to do only one side—this is quite common with people you have treated a few times before. See page 49 for more details.

Assessment

The **assessment** is done to evaluate the energy field. We must find the areas to be treated. As you have learned, the energy field should be in balance at all times. It should feel like the "ball" everywhere throughout the field. When there is an imbalance, it will manifest itself in the form of heat, cold, tingling, or pressure (more or less), or other sensations. I have to note here that Mr. Domancic is against the evaluation or even feeling of the energy, fearing that the inexperienced would have false readings, leading to the wrong treatments. However, this is highly unlikely since the higher self (or subconscious) would still prevent most of the wrong treatments. The same subconscious, according to Mr. Domancic, will do the treatment anyway, so there is no need to worry. Also, he is quite confident in the modern diagnostics of contemporary medicine, thus relying on what his patients tell him their problems are. "I have headaches," "I have diabetes," or "I have liver cancer" are substantial enough. Most of them bring their medical findings to him. Also, working on the feet at the end will address all the areas we may have missed through a type of energy reflexology. In case you are not familiar with it, reflexology is the manipulation (by hands, knuckles, or other devices) of reflex (or trigger) points on the subject's feet and hands in order to induce changes in the body. Since the entire body is reflected in the feet (such as the spine being the inner arch of the foot, the head is the big toe, the middle of the foot is the kidney, etc.), manipulating those points will affect the corresponding areas of the body. Without any knowledge of those points, we can still help the whole body by directing bioenergy to the entire foot. For more information on reflexology, I recommend my first book: *Biotherapy: A Healing for the 21st Century.*

Treatment

After the assessment comes the actual **treatment**. You should always work your way down from the top of the head to the bottom of the feet. Wherever you have felt the imbalances, those are the areas to be worked on, starting with the ones on the top.

In the Domancic method, it is preferred to work on the head, the heart, and the feet on almost all occasions, regardless of whether those areas are out of balance or not. Those are major energy centers that always benefit from a treatment and will positively influence the entire energy field.

It is not necessary to perform the Domancic method for a full treatment; however, it is hard to ignore the fact that this treatment has worked for a million people. Personally, I can do a full treatment on someone standing up for the entire time, even if it is on a city bus. I have done short, quick treatments in just about any possible situation/ position. However, when I have enough time for a full treatment, I do prefer to include the major elements of the **Domancic method**.

Domancic method

Hold the head/balancing

Start by holding the top of the **head** with your left hand and the back of the head with your right. Hold this position with your hands slightly tense for about a minute and a half. Finish by five or six crossing movements in a circular shape a few inches over the head.

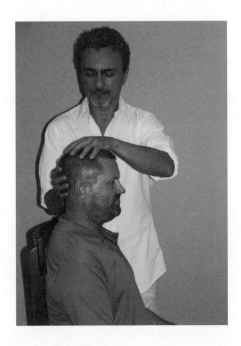

Hold the heart/cleansing

Next comes the holding of the **heart**: left hand on the heart in the front, right hand on the back—both tense. Hold this for a minute and a half as well. Finish by waving off the excess energy with your right hand: stand in front of your subject, and push the energy to the right, then to the left, again to the right, and finally pull it off far to the left and give it a quick shake. It all looks like the wave of a beauty queen with a farther wave to the left. Repeat five to six times.

The head and the heart embrace will produce intense sensations of heat in both of you.

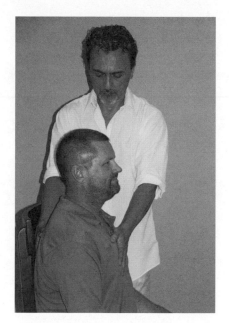

Feet treatment

For the **feet** treatment, your subject has to be in a seated position with his/her legs extended with feet on a chair in front of you. There are three significant movements involving the feet.

For the first one, repeat the same **crossing movements** you have done over the head, except now you have to repeat them for about thirty seconds above the feet (toes).

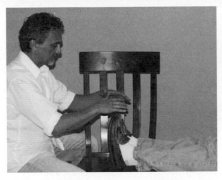
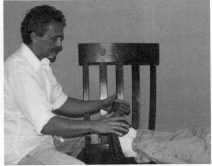

Follow this by **"playing the piano"** with tight fingers shaking as quickly as possible above (or toward) the toes. Continue for thirty seconds. This move may induce intense sensations in the form of tingling in the feet, legs, or even the spine of your subject.

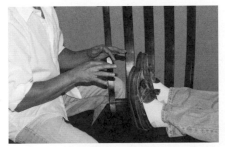
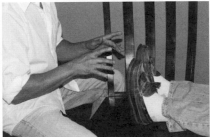

Last, **hold the hands** in the same area above (or toward) the toes with slight tension for around thirty seconds as well. This will also induce the sensation of heat.

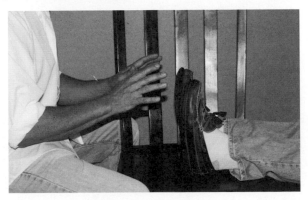

If your subject needs **other treatments** in between these areas, do them in the already predetermined fashion. First, remove the excess energy, then add the needed energy. Work your way down. So if the neck needs a treatment, complete it after you are done with the head and before you work on the heart. If the stomach needs a treatment, do it after you are done with the heart, and so on.

Waving movements

After you are done with the feet, if a positive treatment is needed, finish by **waving movements**—about twenty-five times. In case of a very weak immune system or cancer, you may repeat it forty to fifty times. See page 77 for more details.

Close the energy field/tap

 Have your subject stand up (if he/she is capable), and re-evaluate the energy if needed. After that, do the **crossing movements** and the **finishing tap** (see p. 78). That's it!

A quick procedure

In case of emergency or just not having enough time, a quick treatment may be sufficient. This can be done in sitting or standing (always more preferred) position. In case the subject has to lie down, that is also an acceptable position.

This was my main routine for the longest time:

> Start with the regular habit of crossing hands, followed by the evaluation. Again, from the top of the head to the bottom of the feet, fix each area as it comes. Finish with the usual crossing hands and the final tap.
>
> This is almost as effective as the Domancic routine, just missing some key elements in jump-starting the flow of the energy. However, many times balancing the field itself is enough for the energy to start flowing again.

Sometimes, moving your left hand up in front of the body and at the same time moving the right hand down behind the spine may aid the natural energy flow as well. Lead with the palms of your hands. Repeat five to six times.

An even quicker procedure

In case you only have a few minutes to fix a problem—mainly pain (headaches, shoulder pain, stomachache, and similar) or discomfort (diarrhea, constipation, pressure)—you can just concentrate on the problem area and nothing else. For instance, if it is a headache, just hold the head for a minute at the painful areas, and then pull the energy off. Don't forget to shake your hands off at the end of each move. Repeat until the pain is gone, and you are done. It is still preferred to finish with the crossing moves and a tap. This works for any body part, anywhere and at any time.

11.
Psychokinesis

Have you ever seen the famous t'ai chi (Taiji) and Chi Kung (qigong) masters overpowering their opponents while barely touching them? How about the ones that don't even touch their opponents?! Yes, it is quite possible! Thanks to modern technology, you may view dozens of examples on YouTube or dig out some old footage of Bill Moyers's trip to China, where he personally visits some of those masters. One of them demonstrated his skills by withstanding any punch, push, or throw by literally turning the same power against the opponent in the form of electric shocks. Some of his opponents/students would fly several feet away from the stun! This old man practices in the park every morning at dawn. If one wishes to learn his skills, one should show up early every day and practice with him for three years to demonstrate seriousness. After three years of this, he may actually take a person as his student.

Another master would throw away his opponents even before they would get close to him. Several feet away, their muscles would just give out or twitch uncontrollably. Some of them he would push the other direction as if they hit an invisible wall. His ability, he explains, comes from being proficient in the use of the chi.

Not everyone can perform such incredible feats. Those masters have practiced their energy arts for decades. It takes much discipline and concentration to reach such oneness with the universe. However, some of us are apparently just born that way.

I have been able to move people (perform psychokinesis) for many years without much effort long before I ever learned t'ai chi or Chi Kung. I believe that just about anyone can do the same with some practice and concentration. The question is why? Why should you move someone without touching him/her? Is it because it is totally cool? No denial there! Is it to show off your powers? In a way, yes! If you witness a miracle, you become a believer, right? To most people, psychokinesis is exactly that: a miracle. When a miracle is conceived in one's brain, it may jump-start the healing process even before the actual act of healing began. The mind is so powerful that it can perform its own "miracles" when given the chance.

The practice of psychokinesis serves the purpose of jump-starting the healing process in one's conscious and subconscious mind. Once it happens, it is also a sign of a tremendous exchange of energy between the practitioner and the subject.

When I saw Domancic move and bend people for the first time, I was stunned! Never mind that I could do those things myself, it was still incredible and unbelievable to see it! Many people still don't believe that such things can actually happen. I constantly get comments under my YouTube psychokinesis videos that claim how this is impossible or that this is outright fake. Some people still think the earth is flat. Uri Geller, the psychic phenomenon who can bend spoons and other metal objects, restart old clocks, read minds, and perform other incredible tasks is one of the most studied individuals on the planet. Yet, many people still believe that he is just a magician.

There are some preconceived ideas in us that are hard to break. That is what produces the stunning effects of healing when personally confronted with the real thing. The more people witness such an unusual event, the more powerful the believing and the healing. Once, I pulled back 80 people from about 30 feet away at a t'ai chi demonstration. I was just standing behind them with my hands resting below my belly button without any movement. They all started bending back or even stepping back at almost the same time. These were not just everyday folks—many of them were martial arts masters aware of the existence of the energy. I am sure that, after that one demonstration, most of them became believers!

Performing psychokinesis is relatively easy if you have good imagination and/or visualization. You must concentrate on the energy and not on the individual. The t'ai chi master would say to become the other person—meaning to feel the other person in order to overpower him/her. In our case, we don't have to overpower anyone—we just have to show force. We "see" or "feel" the other person's energy and give it a push or a pull.

There are many ways to move a person. You can push, pull, bend, and so on.

The easiest way to perform psychokinesis is to stand in front of your subject and, after finishing the crossing movements at the very beginning of the treatment, look above his/her head or shoulder (either one), lift your hands up in front and above

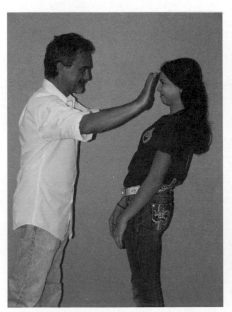
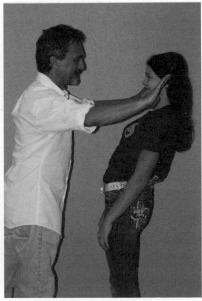

his/her shoulder, and push back on the invisible energy. You should lightly tense your hands and look a bit behind the shoulders—as if you were pushing on the area above and behind them, even though your hands are in the front or above the shoulders. Try not to touch your subject at all. You should visualize the pushing. There may be nothing to see, but we know that the energy is there. The harder you visualize, the easier the person will move.

You may not get it the first time. You may not get every person to move either. Actually, that is quite certain. People with compromised energy fields will be easier to move than the healthy ones. Size doesn't matter. Many times, I have moved people much bigger than myself more easily than smaller people.

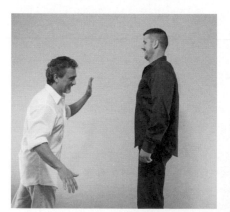
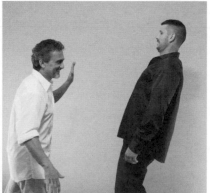
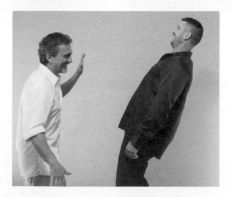

Once you have noticed the person moving backward, keep pushing. You may let your hands go past his/her ears but keep pushing. This is where you show off your powers, creating the perception of superiority and the genuine ability to heal.

Now step to the side, and continue pushing with just one hand.

 This move may turn into a pull: continue the push until you go past the person on the side, and if he/she is bent far enough but still standing, "grab" the energy, and continue your move into a pulling motion behind

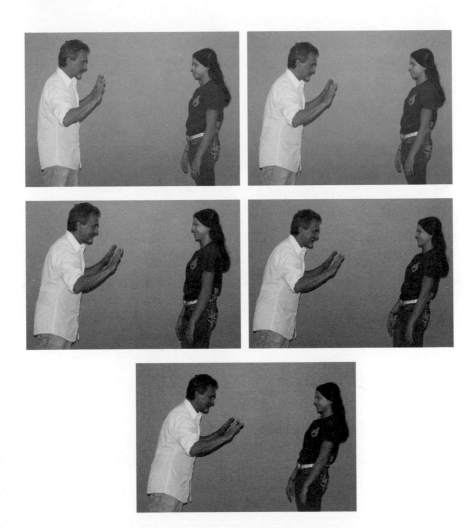

them. If you "play the piano" at the same time, that may enhance the pulling force. You may even step farther away and still have the connection with your subject. The pull can be performed from several feet away.

My favorite psychokinesis technique is to actually start with the pull after I have finished the initial crossing movement behind my client. They can't see me, so they can't say that I made suggestions or that I "hypnotized" them. They just feel the pull. After a lot of practice, you will actually feel yourself grabbing the energy and be able to pull on it.

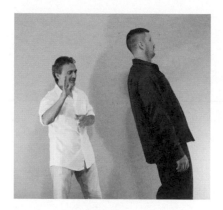 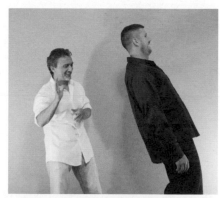

 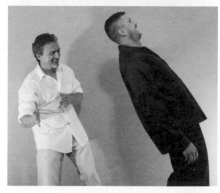

Another favorite of mine is to explore the person's aura in the front and show them how far it goes—usually as far as they can reach. At that point, there is a little bit of resistance—just like playing with a magnet. Most of the time, my subjects feel that sensation, too. At this point, I push on the edge of the "magnet," and with that I can push them backward.

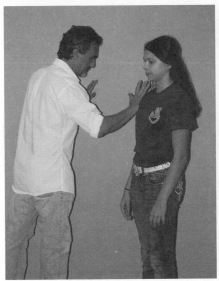 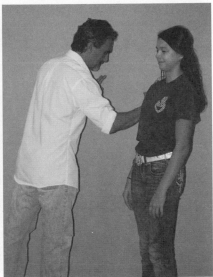

The "nose pull" is also a favorite. I grab at the air a few inches in front of the tip of the subject's nose and slowly pull it forward. You guessed it—they follow forward with their whole body. For the subject, the sensation is usually tingling in the nose and, of course, being pulled forward. It is especially effective with a smaller, fun crowd.

When I perform the nose pull during a lecture—after teaching how to see the energy—I like to point out the connection between my fingertips and the nose, which is intensely visible from the audience, even when I increase the distance to a couple of feet.

Practice on people you know first. See their reaction. See how far you can go and still feel the aura. See how far you can pull that aura. Try it from the side as well: stand next to the person, and push backwards. Don't forget that the aura extends sideways, too.

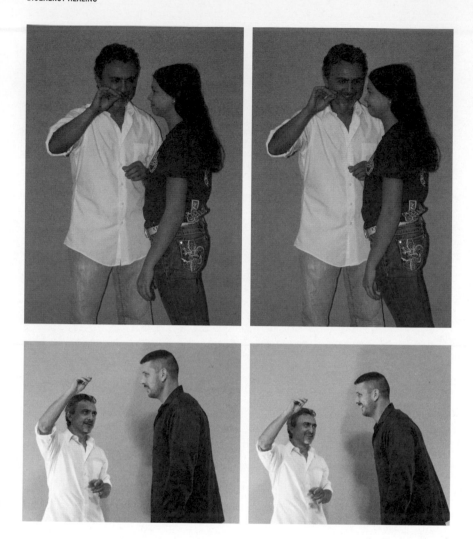

Some people may not move or step back. Some will bend back or forward. Some will sway. Everyone is different to a certain degree. I have noticed that many people will move or get a little wobbly when I get close to them—even before I would start concentrating on moving them. Sometimes I don't even plan on moving them, but I can't help it—it happens spontaneously. A bit freaky for both parties!

Once you have mastered psychokinesis to a point of absolute confidence, you may do it from several feet or several yards away. You may even try to move a few people at the same time.

Ultimately, your goal is not a magic show, but healing. This is just a show of force. You are creating believers. Remember that you don't heal by making fun of people. You heal with love.

I must note here again that the point of the experience is more than just a show when performing psychokinesis. There is such a tremendous amount of energy exchanged between the two parties that some healing processes start instantaneously before the energy worker even begins to address them. More on this later.

12.
Bioenergy Healing Examples and Case Studies

It would be almost impossible to list all illnesses and medical conditions with their corresponding energy treatments. The following are the most common problems that you may encounter. They will also give you an idea on how to proceed when you find yourself facing a somewhat similar task that is not listed below. These case studies may be a bit extreme and don't always illustrate the exact treatment; their purpose is to demonstrate the wide variety of problems and how they can be healed, with sometimes surprising results. They teach you to keep your mind open at all times!

Headaches

As I have mentioned before, bioenergy healing is probably the fastest and most powerful help for headaches of any kind. Unless caused by a physical injury or surgery, headaches will stop in mere minutes of applying this method.

According to the National Headache Foundation, over 45 million Americans suffer from chronic, recurring headaches, and of these,

28 million suffer from migraines. About 20 percent of children and adolescents also experience significant headaches.

There are several types of headaches; in fact, 150 diagnostic headache categories have been established. Among the most common are: tension headaches, migraines, cluster headaches, sinus headaches, and mixed headache syndromes. Some of them are caused by stress; some are caused by tight muscles, while others are caused by diet. It is not always easy to determine the source; however, the treatments will be very similar for all. Obviously, changes in lifestyle may be required for some to stave off future headaches, but the short term effects will be the same for the majority. Most people will respond to this treatment really well, and you may even see some incredible results with some of them:

I had a client twenty years ago who just dropped by my office one day to ask if we treated headaches. "Why, of course we do!" I said. She explained that she had them regularly since she was sixteen—fifty years now. They were of the worst kind: extremely painful with sensitivity to light and sound—a typical migraine. Until that day, the only way she could find relief was to hide in a dark room for several hours and take strong pain medication which made her feel "loopy." She had tried everything by then: different medications, different clinics, and different doctors. Nothing worked. She was desperate—desperate enough to stop at an alternative medical clinic. She was not a believer in alternative healing of any kind. Her husband wouldn't even leave his car; he was so anti-"hocus-pocus." Since all the treatment rooms were occupied, I performed a quick biotherapy on her head right there in the waiting room. She was quite pleased with the result. Her migraine stopped within a few minutes. I told her that we should repeat it a few more times to anchor the energy field in this balanced position. She agreed and came back four more times in the next two weeks. "Are you a believer now?" I asked. "Absolutely!" she replied.

Ten years passed before I received a surprise call from her husband. This time it was a desperate call for help with his wife's arthritis. He said they had tried everything by that point: different medications, different clinics, different doctors, and so on.

I asked her why she never stopped by again after we had worked on her migraine problem. "I never got a headache again!" she answered happily. "Did you tell anybody about your treatments?" I asked. "Oh, no; nobody would believe me!" was her answer. I've heard that so many times.

While this may sound like an extremely good result, it is not uncommon. However, most headaches may come back sooner if the cause is not removed. Stress is the most common root cause of muscle tension, and food sensitivity is close behind. It may seem hard to believe, but headaches may be caused by common foods such as orange juice, mushrooms, or even wheat—not only by the more well-known culprits such as chocolate, coffee, or nicotine.

Full treatment:
- Open the energy field with crossing movements.
- Assessment—examine the energy as usual. Find the areas of imbalance around the head and the rest of the body. Most people will point out the exact location of the headache, making your job a bit easier, although sometimes you will find that the pain is not located in the actual area that is out of balance but is instead somewhere nearby.
- Treatment—hold your left hand on the top of the head, the right hand on the back of the head for a few minutes.

Follow that by holding the hands on the exact location of the headache (if applicable). One hand on the painful spot and the other on the neck is also a desirable option. At this point, ask your subject for feedback. If the pain lessens, continue with the same treatment. In some cases, although very few, it is a deficiency in energy that causes the pain; thus, adding some will stop the pain. If the pain remains, start pulling the excess energy off: from the top of the head to the sides and outward from the shoulders, followed by the same movement in a different path (behind or in the front), so that the entire head is stroked and relieved. After each pass, or at least every other one, make sure to vigorously shake your hands to get rid of the excess energy. It is best if you do this to your side or behind you (see p. 45). It may take only a few passes to stop the pain. However, keep doing it until all the discomfort is gone. Occasionally, the pain may linger on, even after the energy is in balance, but only for a few minutes.

*Note: I have to mention here that the initial holding of the hands on the head serves another purpose. Namely, our own energy will mix with our subject's energy. This in turn will make it much easier and faster to take off the excess energy since our body is already familiar with that same energy and holds on to it effortlessly. This is one of the secrets to the speed of this method.

- Reassessment (if needed)—check if the energy is in balance.
- Waving (if needed)—if lack of energy was the cause. Also, if you performed other treatments in addition to managing the headache.
- Reassessment (if needed)
- Crossing (closing) movements
- Finish (with the double tap)

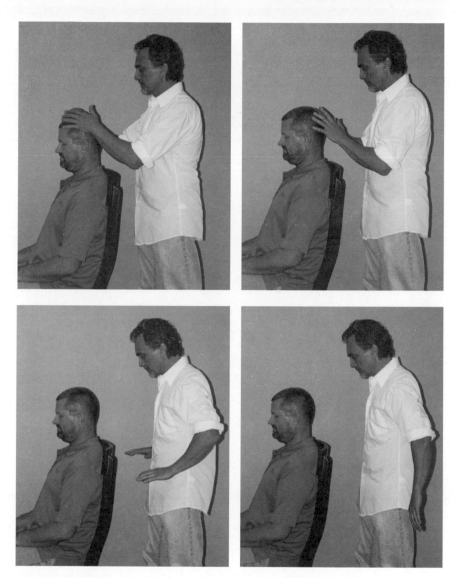

Quick treatment:

Quick treatments may be performed if you only have a short amount of time and/or if you know that only the head needs to be treated.

- Open the energy field with crossing movements.
- Assess the energy around the head (you may skip this part if you know the exact location of the pain), and put your

hands on the painful spots. If there is only one spot, put the other hand on the opposite side of the head. Hold for a minute or two. If the pain stops, you are done. If it is still there, proceed to take off the excess energy. When the pain stops, you are done, or end with:

- Crossing movements
- Close the energy field/tap

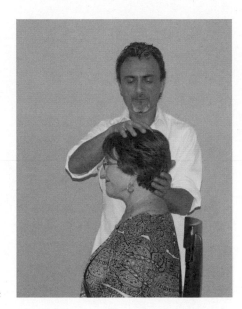

Quick treatment for headache

Pain

There is not one person on this planet who hasn't experienced pain at one point or another during his/her lifetime. It comes in many shapes and forms, but in general, it is divided into two categories: acute and chronic. Most pain can be reduced or outright stopped with the same method that you used for treating headaches. The only difference is the location.

Hold the hand on the painful spot or above it, and if this doesn't help, proceed to drag the excess energy out. Again, pull it off away from the midline and toward the extremities and/or straight out of the field, followed by shaking off the hands. Follow the long (full) or the short (quick) procedure—whichever is applicable. Some pain reacts better to a few waves counterclockwise and then pulling out while other pains may respond to outright grasping and shaking off. Each person is different.

I have stopped arthritic pain with this method, as well as backache, toothache, tennis elbow, knee pain, earache, and other aches and pains. Some pains go away very fast while others take a while. Many times, you treat one pain, and another one stops as well. The next story illustrates how unpredictable bioenergy healing can be:

During my first year in the United States, I stayed in southwest Florida with my uncle for a few months. He was quite a Hungarian cook. One day as he was preparing his favorite paprikash, *he realized that he was missing an ingredient and sent me to the store. As I was driving back, I passed a heavily loaded bicycle on US-41. I was just thinking how crazy that person must be, riding in such a heat, when, out of the corner of my eye, I caught the letter "H," which stands for Hungary. I quickly pulled over and stopped to investigate. As he passed me, I could clearly see the letter and the heavy load. Another hundred yards later, I was able to pull him over by yelling the equivalent of "What's up, dude!" in clear Hungarian. After it was obvious that he was indeed Hungarian, I invited him to follow me the next two miles for a freshly made* paprikash. *Of course, he couldn't resist.*

My uncle was very happy to feed a fellow countryman. As we enjoyed the delicious meal, the bicyclist told us how he got here. His name was Ferenc Maraz, and he was one of two guys who embarked on a round-the-world bicycle trip from Hungary two years earlier. Their journey took them from Europe through Asia, Australia, and most of the United States. They separated a few months before to visit different locations and meet again later on. He told us how many tires they had to change, how many difficult mountain passes they had to climb, and about the many various people they had met. He also complained about his wrists hurting from leaning on the bike for two years.

"Well," I said, "I can help you with that part, if nothing else."

I explained briefly about biotherapy and proceeded to check his energy while my uncle was looking on. As Ferenc was standing in the middle of the room, I walked around him to check all the imbalances in his field. He had a fair amount of them but nothing serious—a bit by his neck and lower back that needed more work, but that was it. I decided to give him a little show and pull him back without him seeing what I did. I did give him a little warning to hang on, but I never expected such a reaction. What followed could be best described by my uncle's own words:

"Well, I was just sitting in my recliner, facing him, as Csongor was standing behind. The next thing I know, this guy's eyes locked up, and he went down, straight as a plank. None of us could react whatsoever. My next thought was: the hell, where are we going to dig a hole for him?! We were just stunned for a very long moment. Then, Csongor did some hocus-pocus on him and he came alive but very groggy. We put him on the sofa, and he fell asleep. It was 6 o'clock in the evening. I didn't think he would ever wake up again. He slept till 8:00 a.m. the next day! Got up like nothing happened! He said he felt like a million dollars and thanked us for our hospitality as he took off after breakfast. I thought he just wanted to run away from this crazy place to save his life, but he did send us a postcard

*two months later from North Carolina to thank us again
and to report that his wrists were still fine!"*

As we can see, this situation was rather extreme. It did happen to me a few times that someone passed out or nearly passed out during my treatment, but that was a very long time ago when I was young, brash, and inexperienced. I tried to fix some people too fast and put in too much energy, which their bodies could not handle at that moment.

Even though I never really got to touch Ferenc's wrists, there was such a tremendous amount of energy that exchanged between us that his entire energy field received an instant "fix." It was such a scary moment that it prompted me to learn to scale back and relax my treatments quite a bit.

This may not happen to many healers, but it is a good story to remember. Please follow the regular procedure and don't be too cocky. A good healer keeps the ego in check.

Back/neck pain

I have to mention this separately because back pain is a whole different ballgame from all the other pains. The spine is part of the central nervous system and also has the role of holding the entire body upright. Since it is supported by the ribs in the thoracic area, it is most vulnerable at the neck (cervical) and the lower back (lumbar area). Today's lifestyle of sitting in the car or in front of the computer or TV and a decrease in exercising has created an epidemic in neck and back pain. Holding our heads even a little bit forward creates a tension in the neck muscles that eventually escalates into pain. Imagine holding a bowling ball in your hand all day—that is what your neck has to do to support your head! If the tension and poor balance persist, eventually your lower back will start hurting from the entire upper body leaning forward. If any one part of your body goes out, the rest will eventually follow. Bad shoes will lead to back pain as well—just like lack of exercise. These are but a few of potentially hundreds of reasons why you may experience back or neck pain.

Bioenergy healing is an effective way to stop some pain in your neck and back; however, lifestyle changes are definitely needed for long-term pain management. Most backaches are primarily physical in nature, meaning that the muscles, joints, bones and nerves are involved, not only the lack of energy flow. This necessitates the use of physical treatments such as chiropractic treatment, massage therapy, physical therapy and exercise. Daily stretching routine, t'ai chi, qigong, and yoga are my favorite back-maintenance exercises, along with weight lifting. If you have never done any of those, make sure you start with a professional trainer.

For ten years, I had the largest exercise class at the local cultural center, teaching t'ai chi. It consistently had 20-25 students; in season, it swelled up to 50. Most of them were seniors with various health issues. It was a good outlet for me, taking me away from seeing individuals all day, while it was also a good advertisement for my regular healing practice. It wasn't only about t'ai chi. We discussed everything related to health on a regular basis: other exercises, diet, positive thinking, and such.

At the beginning of one of those classes, Rose, a shy eighty-something young lady came to me and quietly asked if I could do something about her backache because she was barely able to stand from pain, and she really wanted to exercise that day. She hadn't missed a class in more than two years. I told her I would be happy to oblige and asked her if she could try to stand for a few minutes. By then, most of the students had seen biotherapy in action, and most of them already learned how to feel and see the energy (I made sure that even the beginners learned that by their second class). However, since there were still a few minutes until the start of the class, they were still trickling in through the door. By the time I was done working on Rose's back, I had an audience around me, asking all kinds of questions about energy healing. I only did a quick treatment (see p. 111), but it was enough to reduce the pain and let Rose have her exercise. I hurriedly answered a few questions and proceeded with the class. Apparently that wasn't enough. The result was so astonishing to some of the students that, the next week, there was a line waiting for me, stretched from the front door to the spot where I usually stood in front of the class! They all wanted back treatments.

The quickest solution to the demand was to teach them all how to do it. I had all of them stand in a circle and put their left hands on the neck of the person in front of them and their right hands on the lower back (see p. 110). I stood in line with them. From that point, I led them through the whole procedure. It worked! Many reported amazing pain relief, as if I had worked on them individually. I could definitely feel the energy moving myself. After that day, we finished every class with a group energy healing or a group shoulder rub. You don't often see that many smiling faces!

Full treatment:
- Start with the usual opening of the aura.
- Assess the energy—find the areas of imbalance.
- Hold the head (left hand on top, right hand behind) for a minute and a half.
- Hold the heart (left hand in the front, right hand in the back) for a minute and a half.
- Hold your hands on the painful areas for a few minutes on each spot. If no change, pull the energy off in the already established way (down the spine and out; away from the

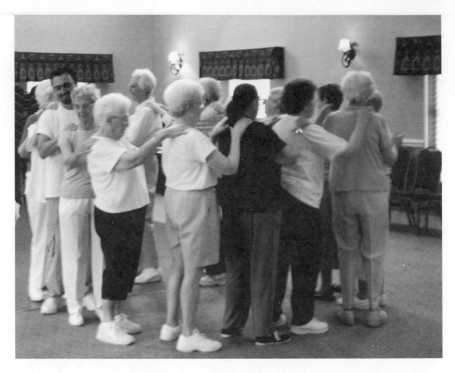

Group energy healing

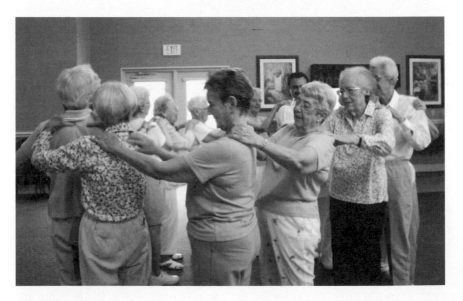

midline; or straight out) until the pain subsides. Pull your hands down the spine a few times at the end to stimulate the energy flow.

- Do the feet routine (spread, play the piano, hold).
- Waving.
- Finish with the closing movements and the tap.

Quick treatment:
- Find the areas of the imbalance (although most of the time people will tell you exactly where it hurts), and hold your hands on them for a few minutes.
- If no change, pull the energy off, straight out and down the spine (mix the two up) until the pain stops or subsides.
- Don't forget to shake the excess energy off.

Note: most of the time obstruction of the energy flow at the neck (especially!) and lower back is the main culprit of one's health issues. Consequently, I like to include a spine treatment in almost all of my quick treatments. After the opening moves, I move my hands up and down the spine to jump-start a bit of a flow. I follow that with holding the neck with my left hand and holding the lower back

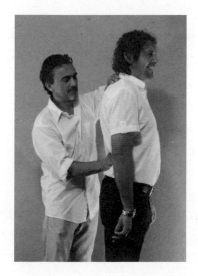

Quick treatment for back pain

with my right hand for at least thirty seconds. This stimulates the energy at those areas and may help with some stagnating currents. It doesn't take much time and is very effective.

Toothache

Everyone who has had one knows how bad a toothache can feel. When it hurts, there is nothing else in the world that matters other than stopping the pain. Your dentist may be miles or days away. There are many painkillers on the market that will help, but then you have to deal with the side effects of those, which may leave you dizzy or loopy or will harm your internal organs. I discovered early on that bioenergy healing can stop most toothaches within minutes. Unfortunately, it won't give you a new tooth, but you will be happy on the way to the dentist!

> *I was just a budding biotherapist, still figuring out my moves, when I stopped by my girlfriend's house one day. Her fourteen-year-old little sister greeted me at the door while holding one hand over her jaw. "Hey, you are the healer. Heal my tooth!" she begged loudly. "Well," I said, "I have no idea how to heal a tooth." She countered: "I know you can stop a headache—just do the same for my tooth!" I couldn't resist her begging and tried what I thought would work. I pulled the energy straight out and threw it away. After about a minute or so of repeating the same move, her eyes opened wide. "It is gone! I can't feel it anymore! You da man!" she yelled. Needless to say, I was very pleased with my performance, and I learned a new move.*

Quick treatment:
- Hold your hand over the painful tooth (slightly tense as always). There is a very small possibility that this would stop the pain. After a couple of minutes, grasp the energy, and pull it

out, shaking your hand off at the end of the move. Repeat until the pain lessens or is completely gone. It is as simple as that!

Sprains

A sprain is damage to a ligament next to a joint caused by trauma or by exceeding the range of motion of the given joint. It can go from a minor injury to a severe rupture of the ligament that may require surgery. The most common sprains are in the ankle and wrist.

My best childhood friend was an ultramarathon runner. He also became one of my first experimental patients. I was just a beginner healer, and most of my friends didn't even believe in "that stuff." Heck, I wasn't sure if I believed in it either. This was before I received any training in biotherapy. He complained of pain in his ankle which was stemming from a sprain he had got during a half marathon run a few weeks prior. He tried everything to stop the pain to no avail.

I wasn't sure of what I was doing, but I first tried just loading up his ankle with energy by holding my hands over the painful spot. Five minutes of that didn't make much of a difference, except for increasing the smirk on his face, so I started pulling the energy out and away from the ankle. Immediately, his facial expression changed to a serious gaze. His pain was diminishing. Five minutes of that and it was gone. Although he has had other issues in his life, for the past quarter of a century, he hasn't had any ankle pain. And I have had a good advertiser ever since!

Quick treatment:
- Hold the ankle for a few minutes with both hands. If there is no change in the level of pain, proceed to pull the energy toward the toes and out, away from the aura. Don't forget to

shake your hands off before returning to the ankle. Continue until the pain is gone. Of course, if there is physical damage, you may not be able to stop the pain all the way, but you can still significantly reduce it.

Tennis elbow

You don't have to be a tennis player to experience tennis elbow. It is a painful condition that is primarily due to repetitive motion or strain on the muscles and tendons of the elbow area. Lateral epicondylitis (or tennis elbow) afflicts the outer elbow area and is basically an acute or chronic inflammation of tendons.

I always found it remarkable how well biotherapy is able to lessen or even diminish this pain since it is more physical in nature. Yet, it works almost every time.

I was at a Christmas party where I knew only a few people, mostly clients. It was a lively crowd from all walks of life, from dental assistants to delivery drivers, from chefs to teachers. I had a deep discussion with one of the guests, debating who was the best tennis player of all time, when, out of the blue, one of my favorite clients arrived, bringing along a doctor and his wife. My client asked me if I could perform one of my quickie magical numbers on the doctor's wife. Coincidentally, she had severe pain stemming from tennis elbow. After a timid laugh, I told them that I don't believe in coincidences. As it turned out, they were big-time tennis players—even having their own tennis court in their backyard—and it was killing them that she couldn't play.

It took me a total of five minutes to explain what I was doing while I was performing a quick treatment on her. The doctor was quite skeptical, even wanting to go get a drink, but I talked him into staying and watching. He couldn't believe it when his wife was able to straighten her arm without pain after such a short session. I could barely contain him from asking me all kinds of questions until the end of the party. His wife received a few more sessions from me in the next two weeks, which included some massage therapy and pressure point therapy for full recovery.

Another episode worth mentioning: a 30-year-old neighbor of mine, who regularly delivered salt for my well-water system, knocked on my door to see if I could unload the 80-pound bags from his van. This was unusual to me since the muscular, former tae kwon do champ was in excellent shape. He complained that he had a severe pain in his elbow and had been unable to lift anything heavy for the past few weeks. He had been to doctors and had tried painkillers, massages, heating gels, cooling gels, and "you name it." Prior to attempting to grab a bag, I suggested he try my magic. He has seen it before, but only at a party, when I pulled back his girlfriend along with a few others without touching them. "I know that you can do stuff, but this is too much for you," he said. Instead of debating the issue, I just grabbed his elbow and proceeded with the treatment. In less than five minutes, he was pain free. "Dude, I can't believe that!" he exclaimed with a stunned face. "I can't feel any of it!" he continued while moving his arm in all directions. "Good," I said. "Now you can unload the van yourself!" To this day, he teases me, saying that I would do anything to avoid lifting the 80-pound bags. However, he has been pain free ever since.

Quick treatment:
- Hold the elbow with one hand and the inside of the elbow with the other for a few minutes. Rarely, the pain may diminish a

bit while you hold. Follow by pulling the energy down the forearm and out through the hand, shaking it off outside the aura. Repeat until the pain is gone. It's that simple!

Bursitis

The bursa is a small sack of the lubricating synovial fluid in a membrane that aids the sliding of muscles and tendons over bones. There are more than 150 in the body. When one becomes inflamed, it leads to a painful condition called bursitis. The continuous movement aggravates the area, stiffens the muscles, and makes it more difficult to treat.

I was asked recently if I did massages on shoulders. A middle-aged gentleman had difficulty moving his arms. The pain was so intense at some movements that he was falling into despair. His happy early retirement from engineering into playing golf and tennis came to an abrupt halt. I was happy to oblige, but when I examined him, I told him that massage would have to wait. Since it was bursitis, I would try some biotherapy on him. He had no idea what I was talking about but would take anything that would help him (a common response by most people new to energy healing). During the first session, his eyes grew wider when he felt all the heat from my hands on his painful shoulder. As soon as I started taking the excess energy off, the feeling changed to coolness and finally to a nearly pain-free calmness. However, his skepticism only went away when I told him that I was also an engineer and explained to him through quantum physics where the energy really came from! We repeated the treatment five more times before he was brave enough for his first golf game. A few sessions later, he was back playing tennis, too.

Quick treatment:

- Hold the shoulder (or wherever the bursitis is located) with both hands, and warm for a couple of minutes. Pull the energy off with both hands, from the shoulder, down the arms, and out the hands. Shake off your hands away from the aura, and repeat until the pain subsides. You may have to repeat more than five sessions for lasting results.

Arthritis

Literally meaning joint inflammation, arthritis affects at least 40 million Americans in one form or another. There are more than 100 different types of arthritis, with the most common being rheumatoid arthritis and osteoarthritis. Not only joints can be affected but other important structures such as bones, muscles, tendons, ligaments, and even internal organs.

I cannot emphasize enough the importance of a healthy alkaline diet and exercise in the long-term treatment of any illness, especially arthritic pain.

Several years ago, after returning to the states following my last encounter with Domancic, I was eager to try out my new knowledge in a group setting. I spread the word that I was back in town and that I would do free lectures every Thursday night along with some healing. I also wrote an article about my Slovenian experience for the local health-magazine, which was enough to create quite a buzz. I had a nice crowd the first Thursday night. After the initial lecture, I proceeded to work on each individual for a few minutes. I couldn't really take my time since everyone wanted to try this "new" treatment. A little old lady sat patiently for the longest time. I asked her to come up and tell me what was bothering her. She shuffled up slowly and told me quietly that she had arthritis in her joints and that her knees were bothering her the most. She enjoyed the lecture very much as this was her first encounter with energy healing. Her quiet voice changed when the treatment began and she started feeling the heat in her achy knees. "Wow, your hands are on fire!" she said. "Are they always like this?!" she asked with bemusement. "Of course," I said jokingly. "Can I take you home?" she asked. Now, this was a common question, to which I usually just smile and say "no."

The treatment was to her satisfaction. She got up and started walking around, trying to feel the pain, but it wasn't there. I got a big smile and a five-dollar tip.

The next week she came back with a few friends. They all listened to the lecture and then patiently waited for their turns for healing. When it was her turn to get up, she just waved it off, saying that she doesn't need this type of treatment. I was stunned! "Why not?" I asked. "You loved it last week." "I still do," she answered, "but I don't need it anymore!" With that, she got up and started dancing. "I feel great! I just came back, so my friends could try you as well. Plus, I ran out of five-dollar bills!"

Full treatment
- Open the energy field
- Hold the head for a minute and a half, then balance
- Hold the heart for a minute and a half, then cleanse
- Concentrate on the painful areas. If they are hot (or for the ones that are), there should be no positive treatment. You may hold your hand on them for a few seconds, but in general, you have to remove the excess energy. If the area is cold, you may proceed to heat it with your hands for about a minute and a half each, followed again by taking off the excess energy. You may ask your subject to try moving the affected joint or area as soon as you are done to see the effects of your treatment.

- No positive treatment is used in most arthritic pain.
- Close the aura and tap

In the case of a chronic phase of arthritis with less warmth and pain in the affected area, you may add warming to it after holding the heart—for about one and a half to two minutes. You may even perform positive treatment to that extremity twenty-five to thirty times. Pull off excess energy if there is pain. Finish in the usual manner of foot therapy and positive therapy (waving) to the body.

Quick treatment
- Open the energy field (you can skip this part for even shorter treatment)
- Hold the painful area for a few seconds (if warm or hot) or a minute (if regular or cold), followed by taking off the excess energy. At this point most people feel cooling or coolness—that is a common feeling when energy is being taken away—accompanied by pain reduction. Continue until pain is gone.
- Close the energy field (can be skipped as well)

Frozen shoulder

I could have included this in the previous section, but there could be many reasons for frozen shoulder other than arthritis. Adhesive capsulitis, the medical name for frozen shoulder, is a painful condition in which the connective tissue around the shoulder joint becomes inflamed and stiff, restricting motion. Whether it is caused by injury, heart disease, diabetes or any other condition, frozen shoulder is no fun. The chronic pain is usually accompanied by restless sleep, further resulting in fatigue and depression.

I have had great success with treating frozen shoulders; although, most of the time I follow the bioenergy treatments with various forms of massage therapy and active stretching.

Dr B. was scheduled for shoulder surgery the following Monday. He couldn't lift his arm more than 30 percent without excruciating pain. His wife heard from the neighbors how I helped them with their backs and talked her husband into trying bioenergy therapy. They had nothing to lose by this point. It was Friday afternoon, and he was my last client for the week. After I explained what I do, I proceeded with my usual energy treatment. Dr. B. felt the energy right away in the form of pleasant warmth and some tingling, which planted a seed of hope in his mind. By the time I was pulling the excess energy off, he was a total believer. I even added a little bit of psychokinesis to the treatment—my favorite move to baffle the medical professionals— which further helped the cause when his arm started moving up by itself. I had only to press on a few trigger points for a full effect. Dr. B. was able to lift his arm to almost 75 percent of its full range of motion after his first visit. Consequently, he canceled his surgery and repeated the treatment a few more times until he experienced full recovery.

One of my favorite treatments happened only about a year ago when a woman approached me at a lecture in Florida. She was a Canadian on a healing vacation at the famous Warm Mineral Springs. She complained that she couldn't lift her arm past her hips for more than two years. I stopped by her apartment soon after the lecture to give her a treatment. Her good friend was watching as the woman's arm was raised to almost shoulder height after only a couple of minutes of energy treatment, and then raised almost to full range of motion after another five minutes of pressure-point treatment. The friend was startled and almost frightened by the time we were done. I had to explain frantically that bioenergy healing is for real and not some kind of devil's work! The next treatment a week later was enough for the woman to experience 100 percent range of motion. We repeated the procedure a few more times for lasting results. (See images on p. 121.)

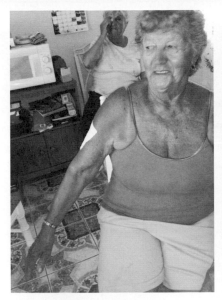
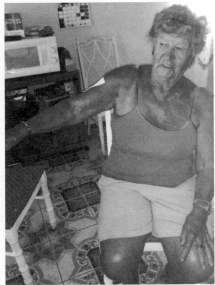
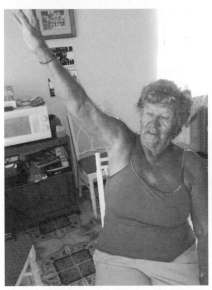
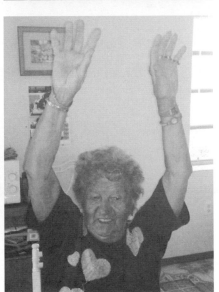

Full treatment
- Check how far your subject can lift his/her arm
- Open the energy field
- Hold the head/balancing

- Hold the neck for about a minute or so until it feels nice and warm. Ask for feedback. If no increase in pain, continue to hold the painful shoulder. Cup your hands around the shoulder, and hold them there for about two minutes. Ask for feedback again. If there is decrease in pain, continue longer as needed. If there is no change in the condition, proceed to pull the energy down the arms and away from the body. Repeat several times, making sure that you cover the entire surface of the shoulder. Now, ask your subject to lift the arm again. Note the difference!
- Hold the heart—cleansing
- Close the energy field/finish with a tap

Quick treatment
- Open the energy field
- Shoulders (follow step in full treatment)
- Close the energy field

Either the full or quick treatment should be repeated at least five times for lasting results. You may do it once a week or every day if you wish—the less time between the treatments, the better.

Carpal tunnel syndrome

Median entrapment neuropathy or carpal tunnel syndrome causes pain, numbness and other symptoms, stemming from the pressure at the wrist on the median nerve. Whether it comes from repetitive motion of the wrist or other genetic or environmental factors, it affects the thumb, index, middle, and the ring fingers, as well as the palm of the hand. To prevent permanent nerve damage and relieve pain, the traditional treatment is to wear wrist splints or inject corticosteroids while, in severe cases, surgery is suggested.

At the comprehensive medical office where I worked at the time, the office manager complained for days about her wrist pain. She was diagnosed with carpal tunnel syndrome before I had a chance to take a look at her hand. By then, she was wearing a wrist splint, which eased the pain a bit, but it prevented her from typing well and made her office tasks difficult to perform. I promised her that I would treat her every day when I had a break for a few minutes. After only one treatment, she felt well enough to take the splint off while, after the fifth session, she declared that she was pain free. We did repeat the treatment once a week, and later, once a month to prevent it from returning. I also gave her exercises to stretch and limber the wrist, which she had to practice every day. Needless to say, she was a good advertisement for the rest of my career in that office!

Quick treatment
- Hold the subject's hand between your hands—palm on palm, with the other hand on the back of the hand, and warm it for a couple of minutes.
- Pull the energy off, starting at the middle of the inside of the forearm, down the hand, and out the fingers—as always, shaking your hand outside the aura.
- Repeat until the pain lessens or is completely gone.

Kidney stones

Renal calculus (or kidney stone) is a small crystal "stone" formed in the kidneys from minerals in the urine. Affecting mostly men, the pain stems from larger stones (we are talking about millimeters here!) that get stuck in the ureter. This will cause spasms and pain in the lower back—just below the ribs, in the abdomen, or in the groin area. It can last several minutes to an hour, and in severe cases, it will cause nausea, fever, vomiting, and blood in the urine. Modern treatments include strong painkillers while severe cases require surgery or shattering of the stones with shock waves.

A couple of weeks ago, my cousin visited for a few days. Since I hadn't seen him for years, I attempted to give him a big bear hug to which he responded with an even bigger bear scream! He was in so much pain from kidney stones that he could barely stand up straight. Years of bad eating habits (fruit, vegetables—what are those?) and high alcohol consumption had finally caught up with him. "Uh, I need your magic!" were his first words.

I had him stand in front of me, so I could check his entire energy field. Sure enough, he was full of imbalances, and his left kidney was literally flaring at me. It was easy to feel the heat coming from it. I proceeded to warm the area even more for a few minutes, and then I went on to pull the energy off, which was followed by a sensation of coolness and pain reduction. He was happy to feel less pain, but we were not done. In the next couple of days, I concentrated on getting the energy moving and balancing the area, hoping that the ureter would relax and let the stone pass. I also taught him "the ultimate energy-enhancing exercise" (see p. 230), which we practiced together at intervals over the next two days. I don't know when the stone may have passed, but by the time his visit was up, he was completely pain free. I even convinced him to try some of my homegrown pineapple and—gasp—a half cup of my vegetable smoothie!

Quick treatment
- Open the energy field
- Examine the field for imbalances
- Hold the painful area (one hand on the back of the kidney—right at the bottom of the ribs—the other in the corresponding area in the front of the body or next to the other hand) for a couple of minutes, warming it.

- Pull the energy straight out; circle counterclockwise and then pull it out; or pull it down the side of the body and then out of the aura
- After the pain subsides, check the aura again
- Finish as usual

Lupus

Lupus was once believed to be caused by the bite of a wolf, which is how it earned its name, the Latin word for the animal. This systemic autoimmune disease can affect any part of the body, resulting in tissue damage and inflammation. Lupus most often troubles the nervous system, the heart, joints, lungs, blood vessels, kidneys, liver, and the skin. It is viciously unpredictable with periods of flare-ups followed by remission. Lupus affects mostly women and can be fatal when affecting the cardiovascular system. Modern medicine treats it with immunosuppressants; however, there is no cure for it.

S. was a serious business woman following a modeling career that was cut short because of excess pain—later diagnosed as caused by lupus. She loved dancing and parties whenever she was pain free, which occurred during relatively short intervals by the time I met her. She heard about me from her neighbor, whose back pain I had successfully treated. She was a wonderful woman—well spoken, with gracious movements, and looked at least ten years younger than her actual age of sixty-something. However, during her flare-ups, her life was miserable; it was so bad that she would not want to leave her bed because of the pain.

I performed bioenergy healing on her at least a half dozen times before she could tell the difference. It was a slow process but well worth it. After the tenth treatment, I started giving her massages as well to speed up the muscle relaxation. Once her pain was manageable, I gave her exercises to strengthen her muscles and suggested changes to her diet (a very similar treatment to the fibromyalgia procedure discussed later in this chapter). Eventually, six months later, she could state that she had no symptoms at all. It was wonderful seeing her dance again!

Full treatment (no shortcuts here, unless you encounter areas of localized pain)

- Open the energy field
- Examine the energy field
- Hold the head for three minutes—balancing
- Hold the heart for a minute and a half—cleansing
- In general, you are supposed to do positive treatment, warming all the problem areas, starting with the spine. Hold the upper spine with your hands, warming for a minute; then repeat on the lower spine. Do at least 30 positives on the spine (pushing the energy up). Warm all other problem areas of the arms one by one for a minute (hands, elbows, etc.), followed by positive therapy on the arms about twenty times. Do the same with the hips, knees, ankles, and wherever else needed, followed by positive therapy on the legs. *Important note*: when subject is in pain during flare-ups, concentrate on the opposite; after the warming, take the excess energy off until pain relief is reached. At those times, you should skip the positive therapy. Finish by closing the field and tapping.
- Feet/spread, play the piano, hold
- Positive therapy at least forty to fifty times
- Close the energy field/tap

PMS

Premenstrual syndrome, which affects about eight out of ten women, is a collection of symptoms that may be both emotional and physical in nature. Although most women experience some bloating or breast tenderness, many experience pain and discomfort severe enough to affect their everyday lives—at least for a few days every month.

I was still in college when I started dabbling in bioenergy healing. At the time, I was devouring anything and everything that had to do with the human energy fields. Right when I was reading a book on pressure points, one of my female friends was complaining of PMS. She was practically in tears from lower abdominal pain. I offered to help with biotherapy, but she was reluctant to try it. Not many people were open to the idea of healing at the time. However, she agreed to try some pressure point therapy, which I hadn't even tried on anyone yet. I found the point halfway between her inner ankle bone and the heel as recommended in the book, and after five minutes of gently massaging the spot, her pain eased. Due to this success, she agreed to try "my magic" as well. I had to improvise since I wasn't sure what to do for her situation, but the magic worked. Her pain vanished, and I had my first happy college customer. Pretty soon, I became very popular with the girls on campus!

Full treatment (long-term treatment for PMS)
- Open the energy field
- Examine the aura
- Hold the head/balancing
- Hold the heart/cleansing
- Positive treatment on the back (pulling energy up) twenty-five times
- One hand on lower back, the other over the uterus (with or without touch). Warm for three to four minutes (add energy).
- "Play the piano" over the uterus for about a minute
- If there is still pain, pull the energy out

- If no pain, balance the energy
- If there was no pain, do the feet and positive therapy (waving)
- If there was pain, you may close the energy after the pulling movements
- Close the energy field/tap

Quick treatment (quick pain-relief procedure)
- Open the energy field
- One hand on lower back, the other over the uterus (with or without touch). Warm for three to four minutes (add energy). If the pain subsides, you are done. If still painful, pull the energy out with the usual procedure.
- Close the energy field

Prostate problems

Given a Greek name that means "protector" or "guardian," the prostate is a bit larger than a walnut when in healthy condition. Its function is to secrete a milky white alkaline fluid that accounts for one half to three quarters of the volume of semen. It also contains smooth muscles that help expel semen during ejaculation. The prostate is not immune to problems. It can be inflamed, enlarged, and is subject to cancer—among other things. Most of these problems occur in older men, but they can appear at younger ages as well.

John, a middle-aged man, walked up to me during the lunch break at one of my seminars, complaining of an enlarged prostate. He had difficulty urinating and had frequent pain that he experienced at any time of the day. He also had problems with intercourse and the related psychological issues. He had a lady friend with him and was embarrassed to ask for help during the lecture, so I set up an appointment with him for another day.

During the first session, he felt heat and tingling as I worked on him—from several inches away. However, there was no improvement in his condition until the fourth or fifth session. We repeated the bioenergetic treatment every week for a total of ten sessions until he could no longer feel any discomfort. A few days after our last session, I received a text message: "Back in business! Thanks, John ;)"

Full treatment
- Open the energy field
- Hold the head/balancing
- Hold the heart/cleansing
- Positive treatment on the back about twenty-five times
- Place one hand on the lower back, the other below the bladder in the front (if too embarrassing or difficult to reach, you may hold the hand a few inches away) and warm for about five minutes. *Note*: If the problem is low sperm count (which has nothing to do with the prostate), you may do the same warming over the testes. **Also note*: Same treatment for impotence.
- If there is pain, pull the energy out until the pain subsides
- Feet/crossing, "play the piano," hold
- Waving
- Close the energy field/tap

Quick treatment
- Open the energy field
- Place one hand on the lower back, the other below the bladder in the front, and warm for about five minutes
- If there is pain, pull the energy out until the pain subsides
- Close the energy field

Infertility

According to the World Health Organization, infertility is a disease of the reproductive system defined by the failure to achieve a clinical pregnancy after 12 months or more of regular unprotected sexual intercourse. Causes (for either sex) range from DNA damage, genetic factors, diabetes, thyroid disorders, adrenal disease, smoking, toxins, and so on. In addition, female infertility can be caused by problems in the Fallopian tube, infections, inability to ovulate, being overweight or underweight, and advanced age. In males, it can be caused by low semen quality, low sperm count, testicular malfunctions, hormone imbalances, blockages, drugs, endocrine problems, radiation, infection, and other reasons. About 10–20 percent of the world population may experience difficulty conceiving. Depending on the problem, there are many different treatments available.

I have been working with infertility issues on occasion for the past 20 years. However, there was a short period of time when five different couples asked for my help. They had all tried conventional medicine (and some of them were still trying) but to no avail. This gave me a chance to find similarities in their conditions and draw some conclusions as to what I should concentrate on. In each of these cases, the infertility was female related. I worked on them for more than two months before I felt that their energies were in perfect balance. (This is also a slow-moving issue, and it takes a long time before results are achieved.) Within the first year, three of the couples conceived, and all three had healthy babies. The fourth couple gave birth to a healthy baby girl another year later, while the fifth unfortunately never conceived. One happy parent—a comedian—suggested that I put "I can get you pregnant" on my business card, but we knew right away that would never fly!

Full treatment (female)
- Open the energy field
- Hold the head/balancing

- Thyroids—warm for one to two minutes, "play the piano" for thirty seconds
- Hold the heart/cleansing
- Back—warm the entire back from neck to lower back in thirty-second increments with both hands. Positive treatment (waving up the back) twenty-five times. I also like to move the energy down a few times at the end—from the head downward to the tailbone.
- Uterus—warm three to four minutes, either with both hands in the front, or with one in the front and the other in the back, or use both methods.
- Feet/crossing, "play the piano," hold
- Waving—about twenty-five times
- Close the energy field/tap

Full treatment (male)
- Open the energy field
- Examine the energy field for imbalances—especially any that may be endocrine related
- Hold the head/balancing
- Hold the heart/cleansing
- Endocrine glands—if any imbalances are found, warm for two to three minutes
- Testes—warm with both hands for four to five minutes from a few inches away
- Feet/crossing, "play the piano," hold
- Waving twenty-five times
- Recheck the energy field for possible leftover imbalances
- Close the energy field
- Tap

Bedwetting

Nighttime urinary incontinence, commonly called bedwetting, is involuntary urination while asleep. It is the most common childhood urologic complaint. Most of it is blamed simply on developmental delay, but a small percentage may be due to physical illness or emotional problems, as well as genetics. Most children should be dry by the age of seven. Other causes for bedwetting (for adults as well) can be from ADHD, alcohol consumption, constipation, caffeine, infection, insufficient antidiuretic hormone, physical abnormalities, psychological issues, sleep apnea, sleepwalking, stress, diabetes, and more. Treatments include medications, counseling, or in some cases, even surgery.

As a young biotherapist, there were many problems out there that I hadn't encountered before. As a way of learning, I tried to gather groups of people with similar issues, and when I had enough of them, I would work on them at the same time, thus drawing conclusions on where to look for imbalances and how to treat them. One of those issues was bedwetting. The word was spreading in my small town about my "magical" abilities, and all of the sudden, I had six kids (ages 4–12) and an adult with bedwetting problems to work on. I worked on them every day for a week and found interesting similarities among them: they all had imbalances in the neck, the solar plexus (both front and back), the bladder (also front and back), and the kidneys. After only one week, six of them had positive results while only the 4-year-old continued with no changes. An additional week of treatments was needed for him and, later on, a repeat for another member of the group. The experiment was a complete success even though I had no previous experiences with the issue. This should serve as an encouragement to all of you when you encounter new obstacles! Needless to say, not only were the kids happy with the results, their parents were outright ecstatic.

Full treatment
- Open the energy field
- Examine the aura
- Hold the head/balancing
- Neck—warm with one hand on the front, one on the back for one to two minutes, balance
- Hold the heart/cleansing
- Solar plexus (basically the mouth of the stomach)—warm for one to two minutes with one hand on the front, one on the back
- Kidneys—warm for one to two minutes
- Feet/crossing, "play the piano," hold
- Waving—about twenty-five times
- Reexamine the aura
- Close the energy field/tap

Addiction

Whether someone is addicted to alcohol, drugs, tobacco, sugar, coffee, exercise, the Internet, or gambling, it is a compulsive behavior with adverse consequences. Obviously, there may be positive addictions (such as running or weight lifting), but not many seek help for those. The typical addict has impaired control over substances or behavior, continued use despite consequences, and of course, denial. Immediate gratification is one of the characteristics of most addictions. Once tolerance is reached, even more of the given substance or behavior is needed to achieve the same effect. When quitting, withdrawal symptoms may include irritability, anxiety, cravings, hallucinations, nausea, headaches, tremors, and cold sweat. Treatments may include therapy/counseling, behavioral self-help groups, or prescriptions.

My teacher warned us many years ago not to engage in addiction treatments, especially drug addictions. However, I was asked so many times to help with those that I succumbed to pressure. One thing is certain—you can't help people unless they decide that they want to stop an addiction and are willing to work on it. There is no miracle solution to addiction! Chemical dependency is extremely hard to treat. It takes various amounts of time to rid the body of different harmful toxins. The general belief is that it takes three weeks for a behavior—whether positive or negative—to take hold. I also believe that we are all subject to addiction—it is in our human nature. Everyone is addicted to something; it's just that some may be lucky to have positive dependence. Thus, in my opinion it is necessary when treating one addiction to find another one (a healthy one this time) to replace the original behavior. For instance, if someone is trying to quit smoking, it is a good countermeasure to start walking, running, or swimming. Not only is it a good sport, but it will speed up the recovery by cleaning the lungs and oxygenating the cells. Still, attending counseling and groups is recommended for full emotional-behavioral mending.

Five years ago, I worked on three neighbors who decided at the same time to quit smoking. It seemed to be an easy task since they had already made the decision and wanted to do it together. They were one another's support group. I worked on them only a handful of times, and the results were very promising. While they all stopped, one of them started again within a month. Two are still nonsmokers today. One is still a runner!

Full treatment
- Open the energy field
- Examine the aura for imbalances
- Hold the head/balancing
- Hold the heart/cleansing (pay more attention to smokers' lungs, with an extra two minutes of warming)

- Liver (for all chemical addictions)—warm for two minutes, then balance
- Kidneys—warm for two minutes, then balance
- Feet/crossing, "play the piano," hold
- Waving
- Recheck the energy field
- Close the energy field/tap

In addition, when withdrawal happens, you can pull the energy down from the top of the shoulders, down the back, and out the tailbone—the same way you would do a quick treatment for high blood pressure (as discussed later in this chapter). Repeat about twenty times. This will calm the body and reduce anxiety.

Obesity

There is a good reason to mention obesity right after addiction. Often, it is caused by an addiction to food. Obesity is becoming a global epidemic. At this moment, two-thirds of Americans are considered overweight while one-third are outright obese. Since 2013, obesity has been classified as a disease by the American Medical Association. A leading preventable cause of death worldwide, it is considered a medical condition in which excess body fat has accumulated to a point that it may have a negative effect on one's health. It reduces life expectancy and increases health problems. One is considered obese when one's body mass index (BMI—weight divided by the square of a person's height) exceeds 30 kg/m². There are exceptions to that rule, as in the case of body builders, but it is accepted as a general measurement. Obesity raises the chance for heart disease, type II diabetes, sleep apnea, cancer, arthritis, and many more diseases. The cases can range from the simple (excessive food intake, not enough physical activity) to the more complicated (genes, endocrine disorders, medications, psychiatric illness). Treatments range from dieting and exercise to medication, gastric bypass surgery, and other procedures.

If I had a dollar for every person I met who needed to lose weight . . . There is no magic bullet or pill or anything else that will miraculously burn fat. It will not happen overnight, no matter what you do. No treatment on this planet will do it by itself. Bioenergy therapy is no exception. It is an excellent tool to help, but more is needed. A person's full, conscious engagement is required 24/7. The real goal should be to become healthy—losing weight will come as a natural side effect. As we know, there are many factors that determine one's health, and all of those should be addressed: mental, emotional, spiritual, and physical. If we put all of those in the ideal range, nature will take over. I could write a separate book on the subject, but there are plenty available. In a nutshell, a healthy adult requires physical exercise (both strength and cardiovascular, as well as stretching; I also recommend energy exercises, such as yoga, t'ai chi, and qigong), a healthy diet (rich in fresh organic vegetables, fruit, nuts, phytonutrients, minerals, herbs, and other alkaline foods, as well as fish), emotional stability (friends, love), mental stability, and a healthy belief system (doesn't matter what you believe in as long as it is a positive belief—you don't have to be religious to benefit). Since energy is part of all of the above, we can positively affect each aspect of the being, thus helping the obesity treatment. However, all the other aspects have to be addressed for the treatment to be successful. Google is a powerful tool—use it! Otherwise, my favorite books for long-term healthy lifestyles as far as diet is concerned are: *The pH Miracle* by Dr. Robert Young and *Conquering Any Disease* by Jeff Primack. They are both easy to follow and good for a lifetime.

I have had too many clients with weight problems to count. The general treatment plan is the same: start with biotherapy, follow with massage therapy (if needed for neuromuscular pain), walking, exercising, and talking about nutrition the entire time. The belief system is strengthened with positive talk and attitude adjustment;

although once the changes start, the positive attitude follows automatically. With this arrangement, thousands of pounds have collectively been dropped!

E. was just one of many who tried my system. The middle-aged woman was about 70 pounds overweight with a very high body fat percentage. She also had anxiety, depression, and other issues that she was dealing with, primarily through counseling and medication. I started seeing her for various pains throughout her body. After the initial biotherapy treatment, I suggested a full lifestyle change as previously described. The first day at the gym didn't go well. She could barely make it up the stairs to the second floor (this wasn't a first either!). We started very slowly with some basic exercises. As the time went by, she became stronger, her cardiovascular fitness got better, and overall, her mood improved. She went from a cranky old lady (as she called herself) to a fit and happy individual, feeling young at heart again. After six months, she was already doing regular bench presses, she was hitting the heavy bag, and she even figured out how to do the speed bag! She was also 50 pounds lighter! One day she confessed that she fell off the wagon and that she craved sugar. First, I scared her by making her hold two 25 pound weights. "This is how heavy you were six months ago. Can you carry it around for a while?" She had tears in her eyes as she put the weights down. It is sometimes easy to forget. We did adjust her diet, so those sugar cravings wouldn't come back. However, if you eat a healthy diet six days a week, it is okay to go for the junk on the seventh—just don't overdo it. E. is now a healthy woman, going for daily walks and to the gym twice a week. She improved her diet, does a lot of healthy cooking, and is overall a happy individual.

Full treatment
- Open the energy field
- Examine the aura
- Hold the head/balancing
- Hold the heart/cleansing
- Warm all the areas where you felt imbalances, especially in the digestive system for about a minute each. During hunger episodes, you may remove the energy from the stomach.
- Feet/crossing, "play the piano," hold
- Waving twenty times
- Recheck the energy field
- Close the energy field/tap

Depression

Depression is a mental-emotional condition of perpetual bad mood and aversion toward activities. It can affect a person's behavior, feelings, thoughts, and sense of well-being. Typical emotions accompanying depression can be feelings of sadness, emptiness, anxiety, hopelessness, worry, helplessness, worthlessness, loneliness, guilt, irritability, restlessness, and so on. There may be physical changes as well, such as loss of interest in activities that were once enjoyable, overeating, loss of appetite, insomnia, too much sleep, fatigue, aches, pains—the list goes on.

Treatments for depression are many—from psychiatric care and drugs to healthy diet, meditation, light therapy, and exercise.

I worked ten years in a comprehensive medical group headed by Dr. Robert Mignone, a medical doctor, psychiatrist, neurologist, acupuncturist and overall nice guy, who was trained at Harvard, Duke, Yale, and Cornell. The place was staffed by psychologists, counselors, an acupuncturist, and myself. I had firsthand experience with depression on a daily basis. I handled mostly cases where depression was an aftermath effect of a physical change due to injury or surgeries gone bad. I was basically doing pain management through bioenergy healing and neuromuscular massage when I noticed just how much a person's mood can change when their pain is lessened or completely gone. I haven't discovered anything new here, but doing it almost every day made it blatantly clear how the mind and the body interact. Today, I still work with several psychologists who refer their patients to me, not only for biotherapy but other modalities, such as massage therapy, exercise, t'ai chi, and qigong. Biotherapy is a wonderful tool in helping to overcome depression, but it is not enough.

My best success story came from forming an exercise group—per the advice of my psychologist friend. She connected five of her female clients (ages 40–72) with me to see if exercise (and the other perks of training with me) would help their condition. Our first meeting at the gym was cordial but cold. All five of them came with their individual problems and had no previous experiences doing any exercise. One of them (the youngest and heaviest) dropped out after the first session. The rest of them stuck it out, although reluctantly at the beginning. I worked on their energy fields, taught them healthy nutrition and dietary habits, and trained them twice a week. By the third month, we concentrated on only diet and exercise. At that point, all four women were already stronger, had lost body fat, and had become real comedians, too! We were all looking forward to the gym days, not only for the exercise but the company as well. They all became good friends and started hanging out after each workout. Other than a few short episodes of low energy, they all live healthier and happier lives now. If you choose bioenergy healing as a future profession, don't forget—mind, body, and spirit are inseparable!

Full treatment (for depression only—if there is pain, treat it accordingly)

- Open the energy field
- Examine the aura
- Hold the head/balancing
- Hold the heart/cleansing
- Feet/crossing, "play the piano," hold
- Waving about 25 times
- Recheck the energy field
- Close the energy field/tap

Stress

Psychologically speaking, stress is a feeling of strain and pressure. It is not necessarily a bad thing. There can be positive stress which may help athletic performance, motivation, reaction, and adaptation. However, excess stress can be outright harmful to the body and overall to the entire being. External stress can be related to the environment (think about driving on a busy road during rush hour); however, internally an individual can create his/her own anxiety and other negative emotions, such as discomfort, pressure, fear, and so on. Continuous stress can be extremely damaging not only to the mind (see Depression on p. 138) but to the body as well (breathing difficulties, tight muscles, cramps, digestive problems, and such). As a matter of fact, according to my teacher, various forms of stress can be blamed for 90 percent of all illnesses.

I talk about positive thinking with all my clients. I actually present my case to them and hope that the positive attitude will rub off. I have been living a stress-free life for many years and it is obvious to all who know me. I mentioned this in previous chapters, but it is so important that I should talk about it again: Everything happens for a reason—whether you think of it as divine or just draw a logical conclusion—and there is something positive in everything that happens (this you can interpret through either the yin-yang correlation or through quantum physics). Thus, if there is a negative event, you *know* there is something positive attached to it. You may not see it right away. You may not see it for years. However, it is enough to know in order to avoid building stress around seemingly negative events. Or, simply master the Zen philosophy that "whatever is . . . *is*." It is not easy being positive all the time. Once in a while you can let go. I do that when someone cuts me off in traffic and drives slow. I know it is nothing personal, so thirty seconds later, it is forgotten.

I run into stressful people all the time—friends, relatives, clients—no one is fully immune. My usual quick fix for them—besides talking to them calmly to turn their minds toward positive thoughts—is lowering their energy in the same manner you would lower blood pressure in the quick treatment method (discussed later in this chapter). Within a few minutes everyone calms down. And if that doesn't work—as you may remember from an earlier chapter—stress is still treatable with hot chocolate!

Full treatment
- Open the energy field
- Examine the aura
- Hold the head/balancing
- Hold the heart/cleansing
- If there is an imbalance at the solar plexus, warm with one hand on it and the other behind the back for one to two minutes
- Feet/crossing, "play the piano," hold
- Waving
- Close the energy field/tap

Note: If there is pain, take care of it accordingly. If the person still feels anxious or stressed, pull the energy off from the top of the shoulders and down (as in lowering high blood pressure) until calm.

Quick treatment
- Open the energy field
- Pull the excess energy off from the top of the shoulders, down the back, and below the tailbone. Shake your hands off outside the aura. Repeat for several minutes until the calming effects take hold.
- Close the energy field/tap

Multiple sclerosis (MS)

Affecting the central nervous system, multiple sclerosis is a mysterious disease that 2.5 million people worldwide have to live with. It is characterized by weakened muscles, blurred vision, tingling, and numbness. Treatments include drugs and physical therapy, which make the symptoms more bearable, but there is no real cure. Bioenergy healing can make a big difference. This treatment also works for Parkinson's disease. Again, this may take more time for long-term improvement than your average treatment.

As a budding biotherapist, I had worked on every member of my family as well as most of my friends. My very first official patient was not far from home either. He was a distant neighbor, a gentleman in his late fifties, just recently stricken with MS. I didn't know much about the illness, but I gave it all I had. I saw him almost daily, not because I knew that that was exactly what I needed to do, but mostly for practice. Also, he was quite a character—he owned the local distillery where most of the town, including my family, made the traditional Hungarian brandy, called Pálinka. He quit drinking many years prior, but he never stopped joking around. As I was practicing my craft, I kept asking him how he felt— where and what kind of sensations. I just wanted a lot of feedback. He would happily provide details, telling me where it was warm, tingly, or where it hurt more or less as the treatments went on.

Our very first session was supposed to be my validation. As I was passing my hands over him, I was waiting for some comments, but he kept quiet. After several minutes of silence, I finally had to ask: "Do you feel something?" "No," he said quietly. Several minutes later, I asked again: "Do you feel something now?" "Still nothing," he said. Getting a little frustrated, a few minutes later, I asked again: "How about now? Do you feel anything at all?" His smile brightened: "I do feel something!" I got excited: "What do you feel?" His smile got extra wide: "I feel a big fart coming!"

Needless to say, that wasn't the answer I was looking for, but it broke the ice (and the silence!) and helped me relax and concentrate on the healing itself—not on my ego. We went on with the treatments for several weeks until he felt stronger and was able to get out of bed and start functioning again. He added massage therapy to his weekly treatments (by somebody else—I didn't know massage at the time) which also helped tremendously.

Full treatment (In this case, this is the only kind of treatment that I recommend; however, you may do quick treatments for localized pain or discomfort.)

- Open the energy field
- Examine the energy field
- Hold the head for three minutes—balance
- Hold the heart for a minute and a half—clean
- In general, you are supposed to do positive treatment for MS, warming all the problem areas, starting with the spine. Hold the upper spine with your hands, warming for a minute, then

repeat on the lower spine. Do at least thirty positives on the spine (pushing the energy up). Warm all other problem areas of the arms one by one for a minute (hands, elbows, etc.), followed by positive therapy on the arms about twenty times. Do the same with the hips, knees, ankles, and wherever else needed, followed by positive therapy on the legs.

- Feet/crossing, "play the piano," hold
- Positive therapy this time for at least forty to fifty times
- Close the energy field/tap

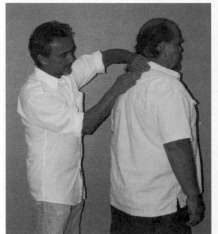
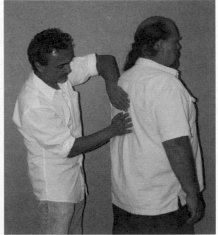

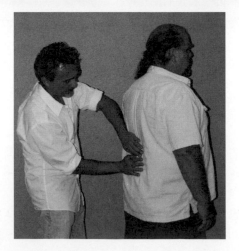

Treating multiple
sclerosis (MS)

Lungs/Asthma/Bronchitis

Treating most lung ailments follow the same routine, except in the case of tumors and cancer (see p. 148). I recommend the long procedure, but the fast may be helpful as well.

Asthma is a chronic inflammatory disease of the airways. It is characterized by airflow obstruction and bronchospasm, with symptoms ranging from wheezing and coughing to chest tightness and shortness of breath. It is thought to be caused by a combination of environmental and genetic factors and is usually triggered by allergens and irritants. About 300 million people worldwide are believed to suffer from asthma. Treatments include inhalers and corticosteroids.

Bronchitis can be acute or chronic and is an inflammation of the mucous membranes of the bronchi—the airways that carry airflow from the trachea into the rest of the lungs. Acute bronchitis is a cough usually caused by viruses and may occur during influenza or common cold. Chronic bronchitis is characterized by a productive cough that lasts for at least three months per year for at least two years. It is a type of chronic obstructive pulmonary disease (COPD) and is usually caused by recurring injury to the airways due to inhaled irritants, such as cigarette smoke, sulfur dioxide, nitrogen dioxide, and others. Treatments vary from anti-inflammatory drugs to inhaled corticosteroids and others.

A classical singer I was treating for bronchitis kept improving after each treatment. We had to repeat the sessions every day since she was in the area for only a week. I treated her neck and head as well. Two weeks later, she sent me an exuberant email to tell me that, not only did she feel better, but she was able to hit some notes that she had struggled with for more than two years. "I can crack crystal again!" she exclaimed happily.

I also work with a band that uses my services a couple of times a year for their singer's chronic bronchitis. They send me an email from wherever they are when the problems start, and I work long distance on him for a couple of treatments until the symptoms disappear. They still contact me even though their singer is not much bothered by bronchitis lately, but now they contact me even if one of them gets a simple cold. They take pleasure in receiving bioenergy treatments. I finally met them last year and had the privilege of enjoying their live music, which is accurately described as "high energy indie folk!" (I will discuss long-distance healing in a later chapter.)

Full treatment

- Open the energy field
- Examine the aura
- Hold the head/balancing
- Heart (Including the lungs. Besides the regular routine, put your left hand on the chest above the bronchial area and the right hand on the back, directly opposite the left. These are about the same positions as when holding the heart. Hold your hands there for three to four minutes, then proceed to clean: left–right–left, pull out and shake off.
- Feet/crossing, "play the piano," hold
- Waving—about twenty-five times
- Reexamine the aura
- Close the energy field/tap

Quick treatment (full treatment is preferred, but it is a good boost between those)

- Open the energy field
- Put your left hand on the chest above the bronchial area and the right hand on the back, directly opposite the left. These are about the same positions as when holding the heart. Hold your hands there for three to four minutes, then proceed to clean (left–right–left, pull out and shake off).
- Close the energy field/tap

Additional moves may be required for other lung ailments such as tumors and cancer, where you may be required to hold your hands on the problem area for several minutes and then "rip" the excess energy out, thus weakening the "alien" energy. Repeat several times until you start getting a more normal reading. These cases may require several treatments and may take a very long time. You should never attempt to work on cancer or tumors on your own without a doctor's supervision. These are serious problems that require serious professional help.

I have noticed that most lung problems are accompanied by an imbalance behind the neck. This is where the energy would travel down the spine and into the lungs as well. An obstruction there would limit the energy the lungs would receive. Check if that area needs work as well.

During the quick treatment, I like to add "energy compression" to the lungs. My hands are in the same positions; however, this time, I move them about a foot or more away from the body, and once I feel the "ball," I start compressing it with each exhalation of my client. I move my hands back to the starting position at inhalation. I continue for about three minutes. It is intriguing to feel the ball getting denser and wider as we go on. As with all ailments, it is hard to predict how many treatments one would need, but at least five are recommended for best results.

Tumors/cysts/cancer

As previously mentioned, treating tumors, cancer, and cysts is a bit more complicated than just a regular treatment. You may imagine those as "aliens," parasites or separate entities within the body. Energetically, they have their own fields within the human energy field.

Contemporary medicine focuses on destroying these "entities" with radiation, chemotherapy, and other means, including physically removing them through surgery. Most of these treatments weaken other parts of the body or the whole body altogether.

In bioenergy treatments the goal is to weaken the energy of these growths while simultaneously strengthening the surrounding energy as well as the energy of the entire body.

Again, remember that you should never attempt to treat any of these ailments by yourself without proper medical care and full consent of the person you are treating. If your subject is already getting medical help, you can still aid the recovery and help maintain a balanced energy.

> *My first encounter with cysts happened at the very beginning of my biotherapy career. I didn't even know what I was doing, but logic dictated to strengthen the energy fields of the body and weaken the energy of the cysts. My first client with this condition was a family friend, who worked as a nurse. She could palpate the cysts in her breast and had the medical background that I was lacking at the time. She had to literally teach me what a cyst was and explain to me how modern medicine treated it. After only the fourth consecutive session, she showed up beaming and declared that they had all disappeared. "Never mind that you don't know what you are doing— keep doing it!" Her encouragement is still echoing in my*

ears and keeps giving me confidence when I encounter a new and unknown challenge!

Not all problems go away that fast; however, it is important not to give up. A woman in her forties contacted me a few years ago about the alarming rate her uterine fibroids were growing. In May of the previous year, an ultrasound showed several of these benign growths, which form from the smooth muscle layer of the uterus, with the biggest being 7 centimeters long. By November of the same year, it was 11 centimeters long. As a result, she was having painful menstruations with excessive bleeding, causing mild anemia. I started working on her in January, and by April (with once a week treatments), her largest fibroid was back to 7 centimeters long. By June, it could not be detected. Sometimes the desired results require time and faith . . .

Full treatment:
- Open the energy field
- Examine the aura
- Hold the head/balancing
- Hold the heart/cleansing
- Positive treatment on the spine about thirty times—important to make the energy flow in the spine
- Find the tumor/cancer/cyst and hold your hand on it (or both hands, or hands on opposite sides of the body—depending on the location). Keep your hand(s) there until really warm—about three minutes. Follow that by the "ripping" movements, actually tearing the "bad" energy out and throwing it away (five to seven times). Warm again for another minute. Repeat a few times. If there is pain, pull the excess energy out.
- Feet/spread, "play the piano," hold

- Waving about forty times
- Close the energy field/tap

Cancer treatment takes a lot of patience and work as well as major lifestyle changes. Since most illnesses occur in an acidic environment, I recommend everyone follow an alkaline lifestyle, especially if they have cancer.

In 2005, I taught a week-long biotherapy seminar in Copenhagen, Denmark. After the daily lectures, I would retreat to my apartment in the picturesque seaside town of Humlebaek. As it turned out, I was only walking distance from Denmark's famous and controversial live-in alternative cancer clinic, headed by a doctor everyone referred to as Finn the Mighty Viking. I knew of the place from my client and dear friend, Betty, who volunteered there for a time as a hypnotherapist and medium. I couldn't pass on the opportunity to visit and examine their work. It was quite a view: little condo type apartments surrounding a grassy courtyard where you could see people of all ages intermingling. There were a lot of kids accompanied by their parents. Everyone looked happy and content. The whole area was surrounded by beautifully maintained gardens and manicured grass. I received a warm welcome and was given a tour of the facilities. I had lunch with the doctor and many of his patients in a community cafeteria and had a chance to discuss the treatments, including the diet program they were implementing. The food was vegetarian, although not without some famous Danish pastries. However, the importance of alkalinity was emphasized quite a bit, along with the importance of love and laughter!

After discussing biotherapy as a cancer treatment, I was asked to talk about it; thus I ended up teaching a lecture to the staff and many of the patients the following night. I went through the usual: a little bit of theory and some practical stuff, such as showing them how to feel and how to see the energy. They wanted to know more. A small twelve-year-old bald-headed boy with giant blue eyes asked me if I could do magic tricks. I said "sure"— not that I know any magic. I lined him up along with a few of his little friends about twenty feet away from me and told them to stand still. They were facing away from me. As they relaxed, I started pulling them back. At first, they didn't know what was going on. They were all wobbling back and forth. Then I yelled at them: "Hey, I told you to stand still!" That's when they realized that they were being pulled. "How did you do that?!" they all asked simultaneously. "Magic!" I responded. I also "pulled" them by their noses, which had the whole room thundering with laughter. Several weeks later, I received a pleasant email from Finn. He had to mention that the kids were still playing with the energy and giggling a lot while pulling each other's noses!

Sadly, Dr. Finn Andersen died in his early eighties in June 2012. The Humlebaek clinic is now an alcoholic treatment center.

Fibromyalgia/chronic fatigue

Fibromyalgia is a collection of symptoms distinguished by chronically painful soft tissue and muscles with characteristic tender spots or trigger points, fatigue, sleep problems, and related depression. It is estimated to affect up to 8 percent of the population, mostly women. "Fibromyalgia" literally means muscle and connective tissue pain. As with other unexplained syndromes, there is no universal treatment or cure. It is treated with prescription medication, behavioral intervention, and exercise.

In my experience, bioenergy healing is enough to stop fibromyalgia pain most of the time. However, for long-term management, a lifestyle change is needed—as you may see from the next example.

> *B., in her late fifties, had been suffering for many years. Pain and fatigue were her daily life. She was sensitive to even the lightest touch. Not only was she hurting all over her body, but she was so tired all the time that she had no energy to do anything, eventually leading to a serious depression. She ended up seeing a psychologist, who was well-versed in acupuncture and complementary medicine in general. He recommended that she visit me for a few treatments and see what happens. Until then, B. would have never considered anything but contemporary medicine.*
>
> *I started out with the standard biotherapy pain management treatments. B. liked it from the very first time. Her pain eased but not for long. The next day she was hurting again. However, even that short time was enough to give her hope. Each consecutive treatment kept the pain away for longer periods of time. After about 5–6 sessions, she was able to tolerate light to moderate touch. At this point, I started massaging her achy muscles, using very light pressure. (You may do this on your clients only if you are a licensed massage therapist.) As the weeks went by, there was less need for energy balancing, and we had more time for massages. Once I was able to apply deeper pressure, I talked B. into coming to the gym three times a week to build up some muscle strength. I clearly*

remember her struggling the first time to even make it up the stairs to the second floor where the gym was located. I started very easy with her, as if I were working with a geriatric first-timer. I had to constantly feed her mind with positive reinforcement to make sure that she would stick to it, even though it was so hard on her weathered body. The progress was slow at the beginning, but within a few weeks, the changes manifested exponentially. In six months, B. was doing full-blown body-building exercises! In the meantime, we adjusted her diet (dropped all processed foods, white sugar, flour, sweeteners, etc.) and started weekly meditation, again for positive reinforcement and long-term results. When B. moved to a 14th floor apartment, we added a routine of climbing the stairs down to the gym and back up after the exercises! At one point, B. forgot about her fibromyalgia.

Fibromyalgia should be treated like other pain, although there is a good possibility that it will take you more time to ease it than regular acute pain. Also, since chronic fatigue usually accompanies this condition, there should be plenty of positive energy treatment to jump-start the energy flow.

Full treatment
- Open the energy field with crossing movements
- Assessment—examine the energy as usual. Find the areas of imbalance around the body. Most people will point out the exact location of their pain, making your job a bit easier, but again, sometimes you will find that the pain is a bit removed from the actual area that is out of imbalance.
- Treatment—same as treating regular pain. Start by holding your hands on the painful spots before moving on.

Occasionally, the pain may linger even after the energy is in balance but only for a short time.

- Reassessment (if needed)—check if the energy is in balance
- Waving (if needed)—if lack of energy was the cause
- Reassessment (if needed)
- Crossing (closing) movements
- Close the energy field/tap

High/low blood pressure and other heart problems

Your heartbeat is a contraction of the heart muscle, which pushes blood through your arteries. This pressure is called "systolic" and should be below 120 mm Hg. "Diastolic" pressure is measured when the heart is at rest and should be under 80 mm Hg. Extreme deviations from this number indicate health problems caused by various factors, such as lack of physical activity, salty diet, smoking, obesity, stress, and others. Those factors should be addressed for long-term heart-health care and are crucial in any treatment.

Uncle Joe (from an earlier story), in his early seventies, was my best advertisement for high blood pressure treatments. An extreme skeptic for energy healing, he was taking medication for his hypertension for more than 30 years. After complaining about it one day, I suggested that he try biotherapy. He had a good laugh about it but ended up letting me work on him. "I am sure it won't hurt," he said. "Go ahead and do your voodoo!"

I only performed the short version of the treatment every day for about a week—with him monitoring his blood pressure several times per day. His initial smirks faded into smiles and full belief when after so many years he was able to get off his medication. His doctor was in disbelief but had to agree that he had no more hypertension. Of course, Uncle Joe, being an old school Hungarian, refused to change his diet or quit drinking and smoking. "Why should I do that?!" he would say. "For the next 30 years of my life?!" and added: "Plus I got you!"

There are several ways to help the heart with bioenergy healing. One is, of course, the typical Domancic method used for either high or low blood pressure. This method strengthens the heart energy.

Full treatment
- Open the energy field (you may assess the energy field if you wish)
- Hold the head for a minute and a half, followed by balancing
- Hold the heart front and back for around three minutes, followed with cleaning
- Feet/crossing, "play the piano," hold
- Positive therapy thirty to forty times
- Close the energy field/tap

Quick treatment
- Open the energy field (assess if you wish)
- Hold the heart front and back followed with cleaning
- For high blood pressure pull down the energy from the top of the shoulders to below the lower back (forming almost a letter Y) and out behind you to get rid of the excess. Repeat ten times. This move is also good to calm a person and reduce stress.
- Balance and finish

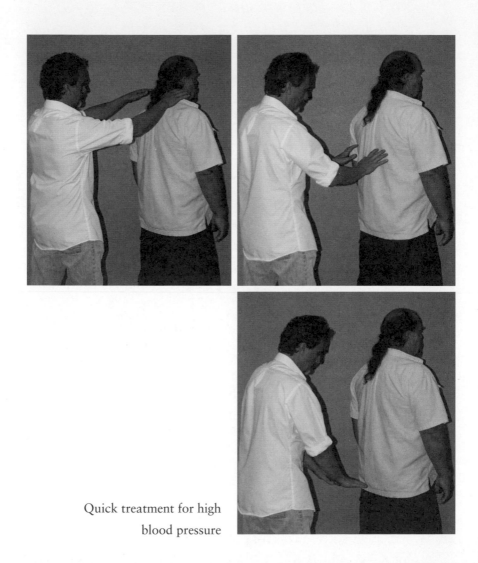

Quick treatment for high
blood pressure

Note: Treating low blood pressure is similar to treating hypertension, except the "Y" movement goes the opposite way. If overdone, your subject may feel as if they had a double espresso!

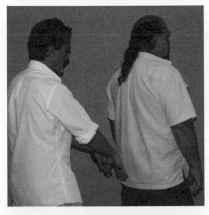
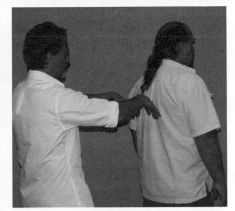
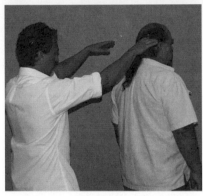

Quick treatment for low
blood pressure

Insomnia

There is nothing worse than the inability to fully rest after a long
day of work! Stress, anxiety, depression, and other factors can affect
your sleep or the ability to fall asleep.

> *Years of insomnia lead Mr. W., a retired attorney, to
> depression. He had tried everything from changing his
> diet to exercise and even passing up his favorite after-
> dinner glass of wine. Nothing seemed to help until his
> daughter took him to a psychiatrist, who, instead of
> writing a prescription, sent him to me. While checking his*

field, I found several imbalances but could not determine the actual cause of his insomnia. I balanced the field and pulled off the excess energy to a point where I could tell that he was relaxing (a few minutes in general). The first treatment was enough for Mr. W. to have a restful sleep. We repeated the treatments four more times for lasting results. His last words to me? "Now you have to bring me coffee every morning to wake me up!"

The quick treatment for hypertension (as described in the section "High/low blood pressure and other heart problems") is also effectual in helping adults to reduce stress and help sleep.

For toddlers and children, however, there is an even better method: have them lie down on their backs and relax in that position. Now perform the opposite of the positive treatment: start with both hands above the head and move them down, leading with the palms of the hands, to down below the bottom of the feet. Now, in a wide angle above the body (roughly outside the aura), go back to above the top of the head and repeat several times. Make sure to shake off the excess energy every other time or so. This procedure weakens the energy field slightly, relaxing it, and helping the body toward a restful sleep. This won't harm the overall energy; however, you shouldn't do it when the immune system is compromised. This method is fine to use with adults as well; it just takes more work to cover larger bodies.

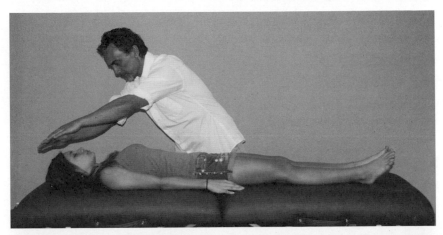

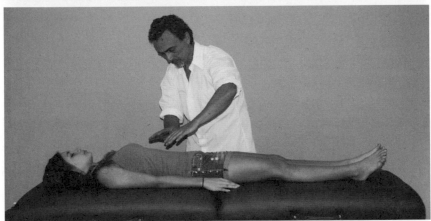

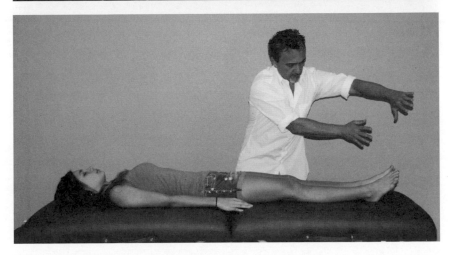

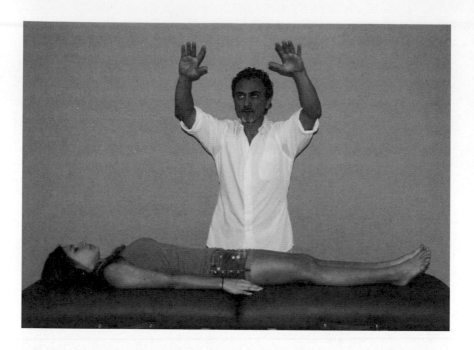

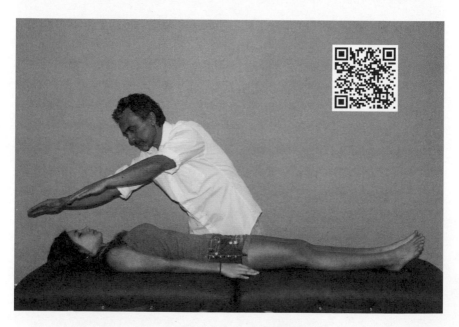

Insomnia treatment for children

Tinnitus

Whether it is caused by neurological damage, allergies, infections, foreign objects in the ear, loud sounds, or stress, tinnitus can be very annoying. It literally means "ringing"—in this case, in the ears. We all hear some sounds in our ears, but for most of us, they are so minimal that we don't pay any attention to them. In the case of tinnitus though, it can be unbearable to the sufferer.

Bioenergy healing is an excellent method for reducing or even stopping the noise—in most cases. I have to add that disclaimer because it doesn't work for everyone. When it does, though, many times even one treatment is enough. However, I have had cases where it made absolutely no difference. It may be due to the specific cause of it, which, if physical in nature, may be too challenging for pure energy work. Either way, it is worth the try!

Many years ago, as newlyweds, my former wife and I stayed over at her aunt's house after a long night of partying. In the morning, the usually upbeat aunt was down and complaining of ringing in her ears. At first we laughed and teased her that she probably had too much to drink, but then she explained that she had experienced this problem for many years and tried everything to stop it but to no avail. My wife suggested that I try biotherapy on her. "Yeah, yeah, your hocus-pocus right?" she said while waving me off and looking the other way. I decided to try it anyway, right then and there, while she was still drinking her morning brew. I just stood up behind her and, after a quick opening of the energy, stuck my fingers in her ears. She started laughing to this move, but remained silent and relaxed for a couple of minutes while I was concentrating on adding energy. As soon as I removed my fingers, her facial expression changed from a mild smile to a total bewilderment. "The ringing is gone!" she said with wide open eyes. "I can't believe it!" she continued while trying to listen to her own ears. "I told you so!" my wife smirked between sips of coffee. Her aunt proceeded to tell us how many years she had suffered and how many different treatments she had tried, both here and in Europe. I knew I had created a new believer and a major advertiser when she proclaimed: "This was the best after-party of my life!"

Full treatment
- Open the energy field
- Hold the head/balancing
- Hold your (slightly tightened) hands over the ears—with or without touching—for a couple of minutes. Ask for feedback. If it is better, continue the same method. If not, continue to the next step: Circle your hands around the ears on each side, moving in the same direction—toward the nose from the bridge and downward—about fifty times. In either case, if the noise increases, proceed to pull the energy out and shake it off. Do it until the noise goes down. Sometimes only the pitch changes, which may still be acceptable. If warming/adding energy was successful, you may increase the intensity with another move: as unpleasant as it may sound, put your forefingers in your subject's ears, and hold them there for a couple of minutes. Make sure that your fingers are tight, so you are adding energy. If the condition is better, you may stop here. If not, proceed to pull the energy out and shake it off. A concentrated move may be achieved by pulling your hands away while your fingers are performing "salting" movements (as if you were salting your food with your fingertips continuously, while moving your hands away; you may also think of it as slowly twisting a twine), followed by shaking the energy off.

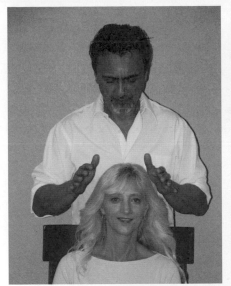
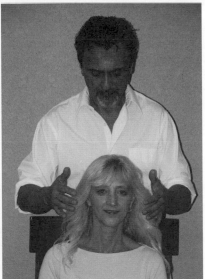
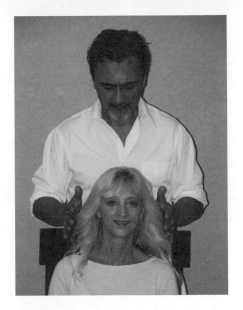

- Hold the head/balancing
- Hold the heart/clean
- Feet/crossing, "play the piano," hold
- Positive
- Close the energy field/tap

Quick treatment
- Open the energy field
- Hold the fingers in the ears (see description in full treatment on p. 162)
- Hold the head/balancing
- Close the energy field

Eyes/vision

Having poor vision in modern times is not considered a major issue. There are glasses for every eye, whether for nearsightedness (myopia), farsightedness (hyperopia), or old eye (presbyopia). Don't want to wear glasses? Try laser eye surgery. There are other types of eye problems that are not as simple, such as glaucoma (increased pressure in the eye that can cause lasting damage if left untreated; in early stages, it may cause gradual loss of peripheral vision); macular degeneration (usually age-related and caused by smoking, high blood pressure, and/or obesity, it causes blurriness or complete loss of central vision); diabetic retinopathy (partial vision loss); cataracts (blurry vision, usually experienced in old age); and others. In many of these cases, energy healing can help tremendously.

A couple of years ago, I treated a woman in her early fifties for MS and fibroid growths in her uterus. She was also legally blind. Since I always treat the entire energy field and not just certain areas, I decided to pay attention to her eyes as well. She wasn't born like that—she lost most of her vision suddenly, five years before I saw her. She had been on disability ever since. Every week, as I worked on her, I paid special attention to her eyes. There were no changes at the beginning. Luckily, I didn't just do the usual five treatments; instead, I continued to work with her for many more. After about twenty sessions, when her fibroid tests came back negative, she noticed that she could see a bit better. This was enough reason to continue. I apologized to her that I couldn't perform Jesus-like miracles, even though I wished that I could. Nevertheless, after a year of treatments, she was able to read street signs. Still not perfect, but it was a big step for her. "Can you imagine," she said, "if I showed up one day at the disability office driving a car?! There would be a lot of explaining to do!"

Full treatment
- Open the energy field
- Examine the field
- Hold the head/balancing
- Hold both hands (slightly tense) in front of the eyes, warming with the palms for three minutes. Circle your hands in front of the person's eyes (your left hand moving clockwise; your right hand moving counterclockwise) about fifty times, then hold hands in front of the eyes again. You may also "play the piano" in front of the eyes for half a minute or place one hand in the front, the other behind the head, also for a minute. Each person is different, and each problem is different. You will have to figure out which one works best for the individual you are working on. *Note*: If eyes are inflamed, pull the energy out, and shake your hands.
- Clean in front of the eyes/balance the entire head
- Hold the heart/balance
- Feet/crossing, "play the piano," hold
- Positive treatment
- Close the energy field/tap

Quick treatment
- Open the energy field
- Perform the eye procedure as described in the full treatment
- Close the energy field

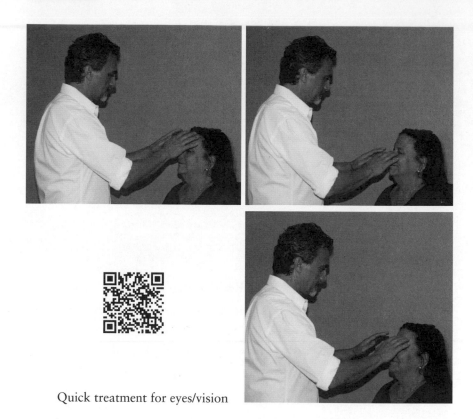

Quick treatment for eyes/vision

Eyes are very delicate and there may be no results for a very long time. However, persistence does pay off sometimes. It is worth the try.

Nose/sinus problems

At one point or another, we all experience a stuffy nose or some sinus issues, such as sinusitis, pain, or even pain in the proximal teeth. The paranasal sinuses are air-filled spaces that surround the nasal cavity. When an allergic inflammation or swelling due to a cold blocks the normal drainage of mucus, the problems appear. Bioenergy treatment can help the drainage, reduce the inflammation, and thus help restore healthy function in the sinuses.

> *I was on a long, boring flight to Budapest when I noticed the woman next to me squirming in her seat and covering*

her face with both hands. She was obviously in distress, but all I could guess was that she may have had a loss in the family or some depression issues. I finally asked her what was wrong, to which she replied that she wasn't sure—her sinuses were killing her and, at the same time, she felt as if she had a toothache. I suggested that we try a quick energy treatment. She didn't even wait for me to explain what I'd do, as long as it would ease her pain. I proceeded with my quick sinus pain relief, and within five minutes, she was pain free. Apparently, this was nothing new, and it can happen to many air travelers with sensitive sinuses—the pressure difference can trigger congestion and the resulting pain. She was so excited about the treatment that she asked me to teach her how to do it. That sure took care of the boredom! A week later she ordered my book and became a lifetime sinus fixer.

Full treatment

- Open the energy field
- Hold the head/balancing
- Hold your hand over the nose for two to three minutes, the other hand behind the head (if stuffed nose, hold the bridge of the nose with your thumb on one side and forefinger and middle finger on the other. After a couple of minutes pull the energy down the nose and out of the aura). Now circle both hands on each side of the nose—left hand clockwise, right hand counterclockwise—about fifty times. This is good both for the nose and for the sinuses. If there is still some pain, pull the energy out several times, and shake it off.
- Hold the heart/cleansing
- Feet/crossing, "play the piano," hold
- Close the energy field/tap

Quick treatment
- Hold your hand on the nose (if the nose is the issue), and after two minutes, pull the energy out in the direction from the top of the nose and down. If sinuses are the issue, hold your hands over the sinuses for a few minutes, and then pull the energy out. If not enough, proceed with circling both hands as described in the full treatment on page 167.

Inflammation

Inflammation is the response of vascular tissues to damaging stimuli. It can cause redness, heat, pain, and swelling. It is commonly used as a synonym for infection, but it can happen without it. Inflammation can be acute, but if it is prolonged, it is termed chronic. Each case creates a different biochemical change in the body, thus there is a little bit of difference in treating them.

Recently, I worked on a young man who had been in a motorcycle accident. His left knee was badly injured and required several surgeries, which resulted in a bad infection. When I first saw him, his knee was almost double in size; it was hot and red. A few sessions later, there was a noticeable difference, but the progress wasn't fast enough. It turned out that he must have contracted some infection during the surgery, and the tissue couldn't heal well as a result. An additional surgery removed the infected tissues, but the inflammation would not go away as expected. We continued our sessions a week after the last surgery, and the improvements were more rapid this time. I showed up for our third session when the physical therapist was still there. He measured 88 degrees for bending of the knee at the end of his therapy. I asked him to stay a few more minutes and see if I could improve the angle just by energy work. He agreed and

*was curious about the treatment since he had never seen
it done before. With five minutes of treatment (basically
warming and removing the excess energy), the angle
decreased by seven degrees, meaning that the knee was
able to bend more. All three of us were quite happy with
the result and agreed to go for a motorcycle ride in the
near future!*

Full treatment
- Open the energy field
- Examine the aura
- Hold the head/balancing
- Hold the heart/cleansing
- If local acute inflammation, warm for a couple of minutes, and pull the energy out. There may not be immediate relief— this is a slow process.
- If chronic inflammation, warm the area for a couple of minutes. If the pain increases, pull the energy out.
- Feet/crossing, "play the piano," hold
- Waving
- Close the energy field/tap

Quick treatment
- Warm the area for a few minutes, and pull the energy out until the pain diminishes.

Common cold

The common cold, the most frequent infectious disease, affects the average adult at least twice a year, while a child may get it more than six times. Symptoms may include sneezing, runny nose, sore throat, coughing, and fever. There is no cure for the common cold, but there are many treatments available. Some even say it lasts seven days whether you treat it or not!

As a father, I have seen many cases of the common cold. I have had a strong immune system ever since I started my bioenergy healing career. I can't remember the last time I had a cold. However, my kids were not immune to it in their early ages. Nothing is more frustrating to a parent than a sick child. Naturally, I have always treated my children at the first sign of illness. I have to confess here that the energy healing didn't always bring the wanted results when my family members were concerned, especially my girls. Being too close to each other equalizes our energetic levels, so it is harder to make a difference in their fields. I was pretty successful in helping to open their noses and sinuses, strengthen their immune systems, and making them feel better overall, but it was never fast enough. In my search for the right treatment, I stumbled upon a few substances that help one overcome the cold much faster. One is called propolis, or royal jelly—a bee product very high in antiviral qualities. It is usually dissolved in alcohol in order to be consumable. Naturally I wouldn't give that to kids. However, the other product is plain colloidal silver, which I started giving to them at an early age. It has incredible antibacterial and antiviral properties. I even got a colloidal silver generator, so I could make my own. They are simple devices that use electrolyses with pure silver electrodes immersed in distilled water. The product is microscopic particles of silver, evenly suspended in the distilled water. It has no taste and is easy to swallow. It is not harmful unless you drink gallons of it every day. In conjunction with energy healing, I found it to be the most helpful method, not just with the common cold but any other infectious disease or even for treating wounds. Ever since then, if my girls feel a cold coming on, they ask for what they still call "daddy's medicine!"

Full treatment
- Open the energy field
- Examine the energy field for imbalances
- Hold the head/balancing
- Nose and sinus treatment (see Nose/sinus problems on p. 166)
- Hold the heart/cleansing
- Feet/crossing, "play the piano," hold
- Waving
- Close the energy field/tap

Quick treatment (may not be enough but good for a quick relief of symptoms)
- Open the energy field
- Hold the head/balancing
- Nose and sinus treatment
- Hold the heart/cleansing
- Close the energy field/tap

Pneumonia

Pneumonia is an inflammatory condition caused by infection by bacteria, viruses, or other microorganisms. It affects the microscopic alveoli—the air sacs in the lungs. Symptoms include chest pain, cough, and difficulty breathing. Almost half a billion people worldwide are affected every year, of which about 1 percent dies. Before the advent of antibiotics, pneumonia was one of the deadliest diseases. Today, it is treated with antibiotics (if it is bacterial) and vaccines. However, it is still considered a deadly disease among the very young, the very old, the chronically ill, and those with otherwise compromised immune systems.

Several years ago, right after spending two energizing weeks in Egypt, I was sitting in the gentle Florida sun in front of the crowded Sarasota Whole Foods Market eating a giant salad. I noticed a red-headed woman sitting by herself, trying to do the same. However, she didn't have a table, and she had a hard time balancing her salad along with her napkin while her drink was on the ground. I invited her to my table since I was sitting there by myself. We struck up a conversation right away. She seemed very positive and chatty. I was telling her about my experiences in Egypt—a conversation that began with a discussion of the quality of the local tomatoes. It turned out that she had just come back from the Chinese Wudang Mountains where she practiced t'ai chi for several weeks. I was quite impressed, since I had been teaching the same style of movement for years. That took the conversation even farther. Her name was Amy, and she was also a well-established and well-known chiropractor in the area. As we talked, Amy coughed a few times and held onto her chest. She went on to tell me how she caught pneumonia in China, and she couldn't get rid of it even after two weeks of antibiotics and other treatments. I offered my help, and we met at her office. Right after opening her energy, I noticed that she was very susceptible to the energy treatment. I didn't even try to move her, but her body was already swaying and following my hand's movements. After the first session, she was already feeling better. I don't think we repeated it more than twice before she declared that she felt 100 percent healthy again! It doesn't always work that fast, but bioenergy healing is certainly very effective in treating pneumonia. It is also very effective in making new friends for life!

Full treatment
- Open the energy field
- Examine the energy field to find all imbalances
- Hold the head/balancing

- Hold the heart/cleansing
- Warm the lungs—basically the same position as for the heart, with additional treatments for each lobe—for about two minutes each. Also, another three minutes of warming at the lower end of the lungs (right over the stomach) is recommended.
- Feet/crossing, "play the piano," hold
- Waving (if there is no fever present)
- Close the energy field after rechecking it
- Tap

Quick treatment
- Open the energy field
- Hold the heart—with additional two to three minutes of hold to warm the lungs—and clean
- Close the energy field/tap

Allergies

An allergy is a hypersensitivity disorder of the immune system. Its characteristics include runny nose, red eyes, hives, eczema, asthma attacks, and other symptoms. A normally harmless substance (allergen) can cause a reaction in a sensitive person's immune system that is usually predictable and rapid. Whether it is a mild response to pollen in the air or a more serious reaction to a bee sting, allergies can be quite the nuisance. Treatments include antihistamines, decongestants, steroids and such—each one carrying their own side effects.

Bioenergy healing can strengthen the immune system and sometimes even suppress the histamine reaction simply by allowing the body to be in its natural environment and balance itself.

I have to emphasize again that working on people close to you is harder than on others. One of my stepdaughters was allergic to dog hair, and my giant yellow Labrador was always at her heels. She would turn red, her nose would run, and she just felt miserable. I remember that, the first time I treated her, it was effortless, and her symptoms eased a lot. However, as we got closer and eventually lived in the same house, she became impervious to my allergy treatments. At the same time, all the other people I treated felt better. I still have a couple of clients in California and Canada who call me every year when their allergy seasons start to drain their energy levels. They haven't used medication for more than five years now. Go figure!

Full treatment
- In essence, it is the same treatment that you would follow for the common cold (see Common cold on p. 169). In addition, examine the energy field, and see where it needs more work (most of the time, the lungs will also be affected, in addition to the nose and sinuses).

Indigestion/heartburn

Indigestion (or dyspepsia) is a medical condition characterized by pain in the upper abdomen or the feeling of excessive fullness. Sometimes it is accompanied by belching, bloating, nausea or heartburn, which is pain in the lower chest area. Most frequently it is caused by GERD (gastro-esophageal reflux disease) or gastritis, but it can also come from ulcers or even cancer.

I had several clients with these problems. Most of them needed a significant change in their diets and lifestyles. Following an American diet is basically asking for indigestion and heartburn; hence, the hundreds of commercials for over-the-counter heartburn medication. However, there are always exceptions to the rule:

Several years ago I was contacted by a young European woman who lived on the east coast of the United States and was unable to see me in person. She heard about biotherapy in Croatia and desperately wanted to try it. She had daily heartburns and didn't know what else to try. She didn't fit into the typical heartburn circles: her diet was very healthy; she exercised every day, did yoga, meditation, and overall was the picture of well-being. She also tried to live her life medicine-free. Since she was so far away, I offered long-distance healing to her. I worked on her once a week until her condition improved, and she was able to go back to her regular life. We never found out what caused her distress, even though she experimented with different foods and food combinations. It wasn't the first time that a problem remained a mystery, nor the last.

Full treatment
- Open the energy field
- Examine the aura
- Hold the head/balancing
- Hold the heart/cleansing
- Hold your hand over the area of heartburn/indigestion pain for a couple of minutes. The pain probably won't change from that, but in the case that it does stop, you can stop here. Otherwise, pull the energy out. Sometimes it goes faster if you make a few circles counterclockwise and then pull the energy out. I also found that, in the case of heartburn, I can pull the energy down and then out. Continue until the pain goes away.
- Feet/crossing, "play the piano," hold
- If you had to pull energy out, no waving at the end
- Close the energy field/tap

Quick treatment

- Hold one hand above the painful area, the other on the back; or hold both hands over the painful area. Warm for a couple of minutes and pull the energy out in the same manner as described in the full treatment.

Diarrhea/constipation

We have all experienced diarrhea or constipation at one point or another in our lives. They are no fun: cramping, pain, frequent visits to the bathroom, and dehydration are but a few of the unpleasant experiences. Causes can range from poor diet (including fried food, artificial sugar, and fructose) to infections, and in the case of constipation, dehydration.

It is helpful to know basic anatomy and physiology to understand the energy approach. Peristalsis, the series of contractions that move the food in your intestines, is a slow process. It is timed, so the body can pull out nutrients from the digested food and pull out most of the water in the large intestine. At this stage, it moves clockwise when looking at the belly. In the case of diarrhea, the body hasn't pulled out all the necessary moisture, resulting in a loose mix. Constipation happens when the mix is too dry and hard.

We can turn things around with energy healing. Literally!

> *Several years ago I was a co-leader of a group visiting the ancient energy sites of Egypt. We were warned not to drink the water, but eventually many people succumbed to the "pharaoh's revenge." There were cases virtually every day of severe diarrhea. Using this method saved many stomachs and allowed everyone to visit all of the sites. As noted by one of the graying ladies in the group while we were getting ready to meditate in the great pyramid: "If it weren't for you, I'd be making friends with this empty sarcophagus!"*

Full treatment

- Open the energy field
- Hold the head/balancing
- Hold the heart/cleansing
- Face the individual, and with both of your hands together, start circling around the belly. Make large and fast circles: clockwise in the case of constipation; counterclockwise in the case of diarrhea. Thus, we jump-start the flow of the energy, or we slow it down. Make about 50 circles. Many times, the results are instantaneous.
- Feet/crossing, "play the piano," hold
- Positive
- Close the energy field/tap

Quick treatment
- Open the energy field
- Constipation or diarrhea (see step in full treatment)
- Close the energy field/tap

Alzheimer's disease (AD)/dementia

Named after the German psychiatrist, Alois Alzheimer, Alzheimer's disease (AD) is a form of dementia. It is usually diagnosed in people over the age of 65, although it can occur earlier in life. There are close to 30 million people diagnosed with AD worldwide. The symptoms include short-term memory loss, irritability, confusion, aggression, mood swings, language problems, and long-term memory loss. Eventually, there is a loss of bodily function, which ultimately leads to death. There is no known cure for AD; however, there are many treatments available that slow down the progress. They are all based on proper diet, mental stimulation, and exercise.

I conducted a group exercise for a year at the dementia unit of a local assisted living facility. I remember the first day when all twelve residents were just staring at the emptiness in front of them. I had to stand up and start up the movements for them: lift their arms, assist with their posture, move their bodies, and so on.

Several weeks later, they were already doing them on their own. Not only that, but they would all anxiously await my arrival. A few months later, we were already joking around and teasing each other if someone made a mistake during the exercise. Of course, these were not just plain exercises—I included a lot of qigong and other moves that enhance the energy flow. Since AD is believed to be caused by plaques and tangles in the brain, there is a possibility to jump-start the flow of the energy that may stimulate the breakdown of those. This is just a theory— no known clinical trials have ever been conducted with AD and energy healing. Regardless, I and many other people have seen the difference, even though the result here didn't come from direct bioenergy healing, but rather from enhancing the energy flow through other means.

Working on my great-grandmother's cancer at the beginning of my career also gave me an insight into dementia. In her mideighties, she was becoming more forgetful, and her short-term memory was getting worse by the day. After I started working on her, even though it was really a cancer treatment, we all noticed her improved memory. Since bioenergy healing addresses the whole body and not only parts of it, without really concentrating on it, I had performed my first dementia treatment. One day at a family get-together, she said that she was bored. She wasn't big on watching TV, so my mom suggested that she read more books. She grew up in the times when work and surviving were more important than books, but she liked the idea. My mom, an art teacher and a part-

time librarian at the school, had an unlimited supply for her. Pretty soon, we barely saw her without one in her hands. She would even sit out in front of her house and read as people would go by. In the next few years until the end of her life, she had read all the major classics— many more than she would have ever read if she attended college! Her dementia never reached alarming levels—not even close. She was witty and smart until her last days.

Full treatment
- Open the energy field
- Hold (warm) the top of the head with both hands for two minutes, followed by the regular head treatment; balance at the end
- Hold the heart/cleansing
- Feet/crossing, "play the piano," hold
- Waving about twenty times
- Close the energy field/tap

Quick treatment (I really recommend the full treatment, but this is good enough for in between treatments)
- Open the energy field
- Hold (warm) the head for two minutes, followed by the regular head treatment
- Close the energy field/tap

Vertigo/motion sickness

Unless you are drunk or on drugs, vertigo is a medical condition characterized by a sensation of spinning or loss of balance while stationary. It is not uncommon for it to be associated with postural instability, vomiting, falls, difficulty in walking and even affecting one's thoughts. There may also be some blurred vision and hearing loss linked with the condition. Motion sickness is a major symptom of vertigo and is usually associated with inner-ear problems. Dizziness and lightheadedness are many times accompanied by involuntary eye movements.

I treated many clients with vertigo; however, one stands out more than others. Yet again, in one of my beginner t'ai chi classes, one of my elderly students had a hard time standing straight and relaxed. She explained her long-standing problem with balance and the diagnosis of vertigo. This gave me another chance to show off biotherapy in front of the class. I usually taught everyone to feel and to see the energy by the end of the second class, but I didn't always have the time to actually demonstrate the healing part of it until much later. I asked her to sit in a chair, and I performed my quick treatment on her. She felt a lot of heat and tingling in her head and was happy to relate her experience to the entire class. When I was done, I asked her to stand up and get in the "empty stance"—it was also a good chance for me to emphasize the importance of this stance to the entire class. The so-called "wuji position" is done with your feet spread shoulder-width apart, knees slightly bent, pelvis tucked under, and the upper body straight and relaxed, with the shoulders slightly rounded forward. Technically, this position lets your hips relax, giving you a natural "shock absorber," which also lets you balance better. Studies concluded that t'ai chi and qigong are the best balance-enhancing exercises, surpassing any other modern treatments in efficacy. To the amazement of everyone in the class, especially my subject, she had no more difficulties standing up and holding her balance. This, after only one treatment!

Full treatment
- Open the energy field
- Hold the head for two minutes on the top with both hands, followed by two minutes over the ears. You may also do the ear treatment, where you circle over the ears (clockwise on the right, counterclockwise on the left) about fifty times, with both hands at the same time, in sync. Follow that with the regular head treatment.
- Hold the heart/cleansing
- Feet/crossing, "play the piano," hold
- Waving
- Close the energy field/tap

Quick treatment
- Open the energy field
- Head and ears (see step in full treatment)
- Close the energy field/tap

Hyper-/hypothyroidism

Hyperthyroidism is a condition in which the thyroid gland creates and secretes excessive amounts of the thyroid hormones (T3 and/or T4). Hypothyroidism is the opposite. Thyroid hormones control the metabolic rate (the pace of all processes) for the entire body. Thus, if there is too much, those processes are sped up. Adversely, if there is too little, they will slow down. Either condition can be treated with drugs or surgery.

Some of the symptoms of hyperthyroidism are: increased heart beat, perspiration, irritability, nervousness, anxiety, tremors, difficulty sleeping, muscular weakness, weight loss, and other signs. The most common form of hyperthyroidism is called Grave's Disease.

For hypothyroidism, when the thyroid gland is underactive, the symptoms may include: tiredness, weight gain, intolerance to cold, and in children, it can cause delays in growth and intellectual development. This condition is mainly caused by too little iodine in the diet, but other causes are possible as well.

It is also important to know that the thyroid-stimulating hormone is produced by the pituitary gland (hypophysis).

I have had several clients with hyper- or hypothyroidism. They were all already diagnosed and treated by conventional medicine, so it was important that they all went back for regular checkups to adjust their medication if and when needed. Also, it was important to make dietary changes for all of them, especially adding iodine or kelp for those with a hypo-condition.

K., a mother of two, was otherwise a happy woman. She had wonderful kids (ages one and four), a loving husband, and a beautiful house. However, she was constantly tired and had been battling weight gain for several years. She stopped working when her first child was born but could not catch up with her daily chores. It is not uncommon for a woman to develop temporary thyroid problems after birth, but her problems never went away. She had hormone therapy at the time but was unhappy with the results. She was very open to biotherapy when I explained what it would encompass and open-minded about new dietary habits she would have to get used to. She already had a Vitamix blender and was eager to start drinking natural, organic smoothies. I treated her once a week for several weeks until she felt more energy and was able to declare that she was normal again. Naturally, her whole family felt the difference, and for the first time, she was able to chase the kids around!

Full treatment (same treatment for both)
- Open the energy field
- Hold the head/balancing (this affects the pituitary gland as well)
- Warm the neck with one hand in the front and the other on the back of the neck for three to four minutes
- "Play the piano" with both hands over the thyroid glands (standing in the front and "playing" a bit to the side of the throat) for about twenty seconds, followed by cleaning (balancing)
- Hold the heart/cleansing
- Feet/crossing, "play the piano," hold
- Waving about twenty-five times
- Close the energy field/tap

It is important to have periodic checkups during the course of treatments.

Quick treatment (for an in-between treatments boost)
- Open the energy field
- Warm the neck
- "Play the piano"
- Close the energy field

Diabetes

High blood-sugar levels over a prolonged period of time is a metabolic disease known as diabetes mellitus, or simply diabetes. The symptoms of diabetes include increased thirst, frequent urination, and hunger; long-term problems include stroke, heart disease, damage to the eyes, foot ulcers, and kidney failure. There are three types of diabetes: type 1 (juvenile diabetes) results from the pancreas's inability to produce enough insulin; type 2 (adult onset diabetes) results from insulin resistance, where the cells are unable to respond properly to insulin (usually resulting in a lack of insulin production); and type 3 (gestational diabetes) occurs when pregnant women develop a high blood-glucose level.

Produced by the pancreas, insulin is the main hormone that regulates the uptake of glucose from the blood. Glucose is the principle food for the muscle, liver, adipose tissue, and most of the cells in the body. If there is not enough insulin or the body cannot absorb it, its functions will be limited. The result is persistent high glucose level, poor protein synthesis, and acidosis.

Modern medicine treats diabetes with drugs or direct injection of insulin. In most cases of diabetes 2, proper exercise and diet can reverse the disease. Bioenergy healing was found to greatly affect this condition as well; however, for long-term results the emphasis is on diet and exercise indeed.

I started treating Jane, a sixty-something smiley retiree, for her back pain. Pretty soon, her other problems emerged, namely being extremely overweight and having type 2 diabetes (a relatively mild version, treated with medication, but on the verge of starting insulin therapy). We began with biotherapy, which was soon accompanied by massage therapy for the back. Given that she was a life-long gourmet cook, it was hard to convince her to start a healthier diet, especially to drop sugar and flour from her everyday meals. She was a people-pleaser, known for her incredible pies, and she would cook anything her husband desired. It was a long reeducating process since her cooking art went back several generations (explaining frequent bouts with diabetes on her side of the family). Once her dietary habits improved and her back felt better, I talked her into joining me at the gym. To illustrate her condition, the first few times she had much difficulty even climbing to the second floor where our gym was located (another one of those second-floor gyms!). Fast-forward six months: Jane had lost 60 pounds, ate a healthy diet loaded with fresh fruit and vegetables, used every machine at the gym (even the heavy boxing bag as well as the speed bag!), felt amazing, and had no more symptoms of diabetes! I may have jump-started the process with biotherapy, but the real results came after a full change in her lifestyle.

In a totally different scenario, fifteen years ago, I treated the father of a good friend (and fellow author) who also had back pain and diabetes. In his seventies, he had already been insulin dependent for more than thirty years. The usual treatments and dietary talk ensued, when it came to light that his diet was extremely deficient in minerals. I recommended to his daughter that she order a batch of colloidal minerals and make sure that he drank it every day. Minerals are very important in just about every function of the body. A lack of even one may result in illness. With that and his regular treatments, he was off insulin within six months!

Full treatment
- Open the energy field
- Hold the head/balancing
- Hold the heart/cleansing
- Warm the pancreas in front of the stomach with both hands for three to four minutes. Alternatively, you may hold one hand in the front and one in the back, behind the pancreas. Follow this with "playing the piano" either from the front or both in the front and the back for about a minute. Balance when done.
- Feet/crossing, "play the piano," hold
- Waving about thirty times

- Close the energy field/tap
- Dietary changes and exercise are a must!

Quick treatment (I recommend the full treatment every time. This one is good as an in-between boost):
- Open the energy field
- Pancreas (see step in full treatment)
- Close the energy field

AIDS

AIDS is a disease of the immune system caused by the human immunodeficiency virus (HIV). The symptoms of the disease range from flu-like illness at the early stages to infections and tumors as the immune system gets weaker. Without treatment, the immune system is too weak to fight off even the simplest infections, leading to death. So far, it has caused nearly 40 million deaths worldwide while another 40 million are infected at this time. Treatments include a combination of at least three medications belonging to at least two types of antiretroviral agents (popularly known as "cocktails") as well as various alternative treatments, mainly focusing on diet, vitamins, minerals and cannabis.

Bioenergy healing has been a great tool in strengthening one's immune system. Working with HIV/AIDS is no exception. I unfortunately haven't had many cases of AIDS to give you a definite conclusion, but my teacher has treated a fair share of them and developed a good treatment plan. Following the plan, I could definitely tell the difference in the strength and overall energy of my clients.

Full treatment (strengthening the immune system in general)
- Open the energy field
- Examine the aura
- Hold the head/balancing

- Hold the heart/cleansing
- Back—positive about twenty-five times
- Feet/crossing, "play the piano," hold
- Waving—about twenty-five times
- Reexamine the aura
- Close the energy field/tap

You may treat each additional problem as needed.

Gangrene

A potentially deadly condition, gangrene is characterized by a dead mass of body tissue. It affects mostly people with chronic blood circulatory problems, after injury, or after infection. Primarily caused by reduction in blood supply to the affected tissue, which results in cell death, gangrene's main victims are long-term smokers and diabetics. Treatments include antibiotics, vascular surgery, maggot therapy, or unfortunately, amputation.

"How can something be cured if it is already dead?" you may ask. Well, the logical answer would be that it is not a dead entity but is still part of the body. We already know that energy is everywhere, including gangrenous areas. Once the energy circulates, the rest of the body follows, including the blood. This is not a scientifically backed fact, but it is well-documented:

> *In the early 1980s, my future teacher, Domancic was already a famous healer. Those were the dark ages of energy healing; thus he was under constant attack by the medical community in the former Yugoslavia. The broad charge was practicing medicine without license. However, he wasn't touching anyone, so the whole case was in limbo from the beginning. Nevertheless, Domancic was very eager to show off his healing abilities. He put himself at the mercy of the medical*

community and the media by challenging them to find him a problem that modern medicine could not cure and set up an actual scientific study. So it happened that he received a couple of dozen patients with gangrene in their lower extremities. He had two weeks to make a difference. The media was there, along with the requisite doctors and scientists. Within the first few days, there was already a buzz. The newspapers would show before-and-after pictures of some of the patients' feet, which were already scheduled for amputation, now showing changes in color. By week two, most of them started feeling the difference while their feet started regaining their healthy pink color. At the end of the study, nobody had to go through amputation, and the test was declared a success. Despite the positive results though, nobody had an explanation for what happened or how he did it. We still don't have scientific instruments to measure bioenergy. Either way, Domancic received the respect he deserved, and life went on. It was a good lesson for us, too—nothing is impossible. Now, any time a client asks me: "Is there hope for me?" I answer: "Of course—as long as you are alive!"

Full treatment
- Open the energy field
- Hold the head/balancing
- Hold the heart/cleansing
- Hold hands over the affected area for at least five minutes, warming it. Do not touch unless it is completely dry and wrapped in sterile gauze. Do a minute of "playing the piano." You may also run your hands up and down the affected limb about twenty times to encourage the flow. If there is pain,

you may remove some of the energy and throw it off to the side until pain relief is achieved.

- Feet/crossing, "play the piano," hold
- Waving (if you removed energy, don't do the waving)
- Close the energy field/tap

Quick treatment (recommended only between full treatments as a boost)

- Open the energy field
- Hold hands over the affected area for at least five minutes, warming it. Do not touch unless it is completely dry and wrapped in sterile gauze. Do a minute of "playing the piano." If there is pain, you may remove some of the energy and throw it off to the side until pain relief is achieved.
- Close the energy field/tap

If you run into problems that are not listed in this chapter, don't panic. You won't be the first one. Think rationally, and try to find the energetic solution. Ask the logical questions of whether there is too much energy or too little energy, if there is energy flow, and so on, and you will be able to take on any task. Relax, trust yourself, and the answers will come.

13.
Group Healing

Once you become a proficient and experienced bioenergy healer, you may take on the task of healing more than one individual at the same time. There are two types of group healings: one is when you heal several people at the same time—even hundreds; the other is when you work on one individual at a time while surrounded by many more.

Let's face it—the first type is out of reach for most people, even for the most experienced healers. It takes more than just energy to heal large crowds. It requires a special gift, skill, and charisma. If Mick Jagger were a healer, he could certainly do it! That said, don't be discouraged. You can practice with smaller groups (for instance, at a lecture) and grow to larger ones at your own pace.

The second type of group healing is more personal, realistic, and accessible to an established biotherapist. In this setting, while you work on one individual, everyone else is sitting around and watching. There are several factors playing to your advantage here, as well as to the advantage of the people waiting to be healed:

- First of all, there are more people; thus there is more energy. The individual energy field's tendency (at a subconscious level, of course) is to pick up energy when it needs it. During the healing session, as you know, a lot of energy is taken out of an individual's energy field, especially in the case of pain.

This energy is not "bad" or "dirty" or "sick"—just excess. The discarded energy is freely available to the individuals sitting around. If their bodies need it, they will pull them in like magnets. It is recommended for the audience to keep their hands separated and turned up, so they will "open up" to the incoming energy. The best position is to keep their hands palms-up, resting on their legs while sitting.

- Second, there will always be skeptics or desperate individuals in a dire need of some positive evidence. Not everyone will react to the energy healing session in a positive manner right away. However, in the group setting, there will always be those who react exceptionally. Their pain vanishes within minutes; they can move better; they can stand up easier; they smile for the first time in ages; and especially, they move around while governed by this invisible energy. This all happens in front of everyone. Obviously, if you see something so astonishing with your own eyes, you become a believer, right? Consequently, if you become a believer, your energy opens up more easily to the healing process. It may jump-start the process even before the healer's intervention. Never underestimate the power of belief!

- Third, in a group setting you can educate several people at the same time. Bioenergy healing is still not well known in most of the Western world. Instead of explaining to each individual what you are doing, you have to do it only once in front of a whole group. Also, you may talk during the sessions and provide additional explanations for your movements at any given moment. You may also answer questions if you want, further educating your audience and promoting belief in the technique.

One of America's and the world's most mineral-rich waters is only twenty minutes away from my house. Warm Mineral Springs has a year-round temperature of

87 degrees Fahrenheit and contains fifty-one minerals. Its healing powers are legendary. The 240-foot-deep salty lake is visited by more than 100,000 people a year. It is also one of my favorite places for group healing. At one time, I was holding sessions there at least once a week. (I also taught bioenergy healing to future practitioners once a month.)

Since there are visitors to the lake from all parts of the world, some are familiar with one type or another of energy healing while others are not. This prompted me to include a lecture about it for the first part of the sessions, usually about half an hour (longer if it was a bigger crowd). I had anywhere from five to over thirty listeners each time. With soothing music in the background and the smell of sulfur from their bodies, chairs set in semicircle, and a tropical view from the large windows, it was the perfect setting. I would explain briefly the history of energy healing, especially biotherapy, followed by a quick lecture in quantum physics for the science-minded. I would also teach the audience to feel the energy, to offer some evidence to their skeptical minds. By now, they were ready to see some action. Depending on how many people I had to work on, I would take my time with the first few and push and/or pull them a little to show off my psychokinetic abilities (again working on the mind-energy). By now, everyone's energy would be working with me. Many people just sitting there would feel the tingling sensation in their hands or even in their problem areas. Since I was limited by time, I wouldn't always be able to work on everyone individually. If there were still people waiting at the end, I would do the "other" group healing for a few minutes on all of them at the same time. It may not have been enough for some, but under the circumstances, it worked really well. By the end, they would all be believers. We all left these sessions in good spirits and with big smiles on our faces.

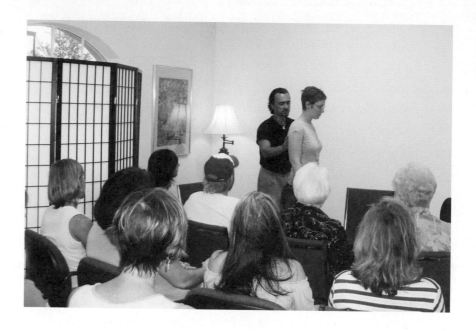

The fast-paced lifestyle in the United States limits these group sessions (and individual healings as well) to only one or two a week. There are very few people who could commit to more than that during the day and not many are up for night sessions. However, in the former Yugoslavia, I was able to follow a different plan. The Domancic method has an interesting premise that follows a natural rhythm. We have been governed by the days of the week since a very young age. Monday is usually a low-energy day whether we go to school or to work. Tuesday is somewhat better, but our energy doesn't reach its height until Wednesday or Thursday. Friday is nearly the weekend, so we tend to wind down. We are the most relaxed during the weekend. With this in mind, working on the energy field every day of the work-week would be the most effectual. Starting on Monday, we get a slow start, checking the energy and balancing it gently. The body probably won't be able to hold on to that balance and will tend to go back to almost where it was before. However, Tuesday, we put it in balance again, and this time it may hold on to it a bit longer. By Wednesday, both the therapist and the patient are on a weekly high, and the treatment can get to its maximum. Now the body would hold on to the energy even better. Thursday is a full-blown session as well while Friday is mostly icing on the cake. The theory is that five days of constant balancing eventually makes the body get used to it, and it will stay balanced. In severe cases, another week of treatments is needed, which can be repeated again later on.

One additional positive factor in group sessions is communication between attendees. Not only do they see the results in each other, but they start talking more and exchanging experiences about their healing as well as other contributing factors to their health, such as diet and exercise. At least in my group sessions, I try to cover all aspects of healthy living including the above, coupled with positive thinking and the universal pursuit of happiness.

If you ever want to perform group healing, take your time to think it over. What would the attendees expect? How would you conduct yourself? What would be the perfect setting? What would compose pleasant surroundings (both sights and sounds)? You would certainly want quiet, relaxing music in the background— something that soothes the soul. For the eyes, pleasant colors on the wall, maybe some nice paintings to look at, but nothing that would take one's attention away from the healing itself. Healthy lush green plants would certainly raise the energy level as well. Infusion of aromatic essential oils may start the healing as soon as one enters the room. Anything that you would consider for a relaxing private room would work for a group therapy area as well.

Group healing sessions are exhausting for the practitioner. There are no breaks, just a lot of standing, moving, and talking. The questions from the spectators never stop. You have to be in top shape at all times. However, the payoff is beyond belief—and I don't mean monetary. Your energy is constantly flowing—even more than during the regular treatments. Just as the audience experiences a bigger energy "high" during the group setting, so does the healer. Yes, you will be worn out, but you will also get your energy to incredible levels!

14.
Healing Animals and Plants

As everything in nature consists of energy, animals and plants are no exception. They too are governed by natural laws, including the flow of energy in order to achieve balance.

Animals

I have been asked many times to work on animals—not only on pets but wild animals in rescue and rehab centers as well. I have worked on dogs, cats, horses, rabbits, swans, doves, parrots, and even snakes. It was a bit of a challenge at the beginning until I realized that the animals' energy was the same as with humans. Animals won't tell you directly what their problems are, but checking the field will give you a good idea of what to work on. Sometimes it is even better that way since there is no interference from a talking (or suggesting) client.

One of my first regular canine "clients" was Cheyenne, my own Labrador retriever. As she was getting old, she developed some arthritis and got to a point where she could barely get up. Her morning routine of running out and getting the newspaper became quite a task. What was once a quick sprint in and out now looked more like a crawl governed by stiff joints and pain. I decided to give bioenergy healing a try to see if I could make her feel better. In addition, every morning before getting up, she would receive a short massage, especially around her hip and shoulder joints. Within a few days, this became the new routine. She wouldn't even move before receiving her morning rubdown, but then she would spring up and happily go down the driveway for the paper, followed by breakfast. Once the energy healing became a routine as well, she was once again joining us on our daily walks and even did some light jogging once in a while.

I noticed some imbalances in her energy field that were quite numerous. At the next yearly checkup, they turned out to be tumors. The vet didn't estimate much time for her to live—she was too old for any treatments to reasonably be considered. She was an old grandma—which reminded me of my own great-grandmother who lived so much longer than predicted after I started working on her. This was enough for me to keep working on Cheyenne. She lived another painless year and died peacefully in my arms.

When working on animals, the biggest difference from humans is the variety of sizes. Sure, they don't talk, but nor do babies, and we can still give them a good treatment. The length of the treatment may be affected by the size but not as much as you would think. The size of the energy field around animals is also proportionate to their bodies, forming a modified egg shape around them—"modified" since I am putting all of them into one category. Obviously a snake's energy field will look quite unlike an egg while a gorilla's will look very much like a human energy field (not that I have ever worked on a gorilla). The animals you may encounter most frequently for energy work are common pets: dogs, cats, and maybe horses.

The easiest mindset when working on an animal is to look at it the same way you would look at a human—except that the spine is horizontal. However, the energy still follows the same routes. The central nervous system is still the most susceptible to the energy and the changes in it. The neck and the lower back are still crucial points.

Opening the energy field is done with the same crisscross movements, as well as the examining of the aura—going from head to toe. Once the imbalances are found, the same movements apply as with humans.

Working with horses may be a challenge because of the dimensions. Forget about the crisscross moves—you wouldn't be able to do it from standing in one spot any way (unless you're Shaquille O'Neal, perhaps). Also, horses are very sensitive animals and if you are not familiar with them or with handling them, I wouldn't recommend working with them. However, at the same time, they are intelligent and fascinating creatures that really appreciate good energy work or a good massage!

> *Years ago I was taking my daughters horseback riding at a local stable. During one of the rides, I noticed my horse slightly favoring his left hind leg. He didn't act upset, but I could "feel" that he wasn't right. After the ride, while we were all brushing off our horses, I decided to check my ride's energy. I didn't go into a major checkup, just the area I suspected of having imbalances—the left hip and down the leg. Sure enough, I found a spot—on what would be the gluteus maximus on a human—that was out of balance. It emitted heat and was easy to feel. After a quick relief of energy, there was a bit of leftover that I decided to massage out. Whoa! As soon as I touched the spot, the horse jerked aside. I tried again—this time more gently and was able to slowly massage the spot out. By the time I was done, my stallion was in horse*

heaven. At that point, the owner of the stable had shown up and saw the horse standing with a loose, relaxed left leg. She asked what I did to it, to which I explained as well as I could about the energy and the massage. "This horse was noticeably having problems before, and now he is like new!" she beamed. "Can you do it with the rest of them?" she asked. "I have a stable full for you!" I was happy to work on them. It was a new experience for me and a good opportunity to feel so many horses' energy fields and thus have a real scientific evaluation—if not fully scientific, at least a statistical assessment! These animals are indeed very sensitive to energy healing. They feel it well and respond kindly. Many of them needed massages, too, for tight muscles and the occasional knot. They are very sensitive to touch as well—much more so than people. It takes a lot of patience to work with them, but the results are well worth the effort. We spent a lot of time at the stables. While my girls were becoming good riders, I spent less time in the saddle and more time working on my new "patients" with names such as Cabbie, Dixie, Prince, Roper, and Misty. Eventually, when I would show up in the stables, all of the horses' heads would turn toward me. I could almost hear their telepathic calls: "Pick me, pick me!"

Plants

Working with plants should be a relatively easy task. Their energy is more primitive, yet they respond well. Chlorophyll, the green pigment in plants, a very important biomolecule critical in photosynthesis, is interestingly very similar to our red blood cells (vegetarians rejoice!). Thus, we are more closely related to plants on some basic level than we tend to think.

We all know someone with a "green thumb"—people who have the nicest gardens, greenest grass, and luscious flowers growing everywhere. It is not uncommon to hear them talk to their plants or even sing to them. Sound crazy? There is more to it than you think. You can try a simple experiment at your home. Buy two plants of the same type and size, and give them the same amount of light, water, and nutrition. Separate them some distance. Be nice and talk to one of them every day ("Hi baby, how are you? You are so beautiful" etc.) while ignoring the other. See what happens within days of doing this. The plant that you verbally loved will flourish. The other one will be slower in development. If you want more drastic display of differences, give all your anger and negative thoughts to the other plant. What do you think will happen to it? The results will astonish you. Of course, by now you know enough about the energy to understand why this phenomenon takes place. You may try all of the above without talk and just use your energy alone. Energize one of the plants, ignore the other, and see what happens. Try it on a larger scale!

I always had a green thumb until I got too busy to take care of my garden and started ignoring it altogether. Needless to say, there wasn't much to reap after a few years of neglect. I stopped even thinking about the energy aspect of my garden until one of my clients—an attorney, nonetheless—asked me if I could work on his plants. He tried growing vines on the outside walls of his house, which really put his patience to test. He tried automatic water dripping, plant foods, even talking to his plants, but nothing changed. They all stopped growing at one point. I took it as a personal challenge and a good way to develop new skills (and be paid for it!). I showed up once a week to do plant therapy. At the beginning, I sat with each vine for several minutes and concentrated on jump-

starting an energy flow from the roots up. They seemed to have responded well—there was a considerable change from one week to the next. After the third session, I decided to try something new: distance healing on plants. As a matter of fact, this wasn't the typical long-distance healing (LDH) described in the next chapter since I was doing it on the premises, but there was still some distance to most of the plants.

I sat down in the middle of the backyard on a comfortable lawn chair and went into a deep meditation. It was relatively easy. The weather was perfect in the Florida spring with a light breeze and T-shirt-wearing temperature, some songbirds busy in the distance, and no visible alligators in the small canal behind the house. Once I reached my "level," I visualized and went to work on each plant around the house. I didn't have to be there with them physically since the energy travels any distance instantly, and I was close anyway. I could clearly see each plant's energy and could make it grow and flow any which way I could visualize it. I saw the energy going deep into the ground for more root power as well as going up and branching for more greens, more leaves, and more chlorophyll.

If I had any doubts about this system working, they all went away with the next visit. Each of the vines got bigger and bushier within a week! An exotic tree on the premises that had succumbed to the only frosty night in the region a couple of months before was now sprouting a new branch! From then on, I was there once a week until the place turned into a jungle. If you ever have any fears about your energy performance, work on plants!

Bioenergy healing on plants is definitely different from working on humans or animals. They don't speak—just like animals—but you can still feel the imbalances in their systems. Obviously, it would be hard to check the energy field around a giant oak tree (although you can see the energy around it if you are some distance away), but you can still load it up with energy. A smaller plant will be easier to work on. You can open the energy as you did before, and just concentrate on the simple connection between "heaven and earth"—the energy flow from the bottom to the top and back. As long as there are no physical or energetic breaks between those two, it will be easy to start up the flow. As with humans, it is important for the plant to get the right amount of water and nutrition as well. The energy healing alone is not enough. However, the results will be quite obvious even to the naked eye. Enjoy your new green thumb!

Cleve Backster, a leading polygraph expert whose Backster Zone Comparison Test is the worldwide standard for lie detection, had a life changing event on the morning of February 2, 1966. At that moment, he threatened his test subject's well-being. The subject had responded electrochemically to his threat. The weird part? His subject was a plant!

Since then, Backster has conducted hundreds of experiments, demonstrating not only that live plants respond to our emotions and intents, but so do severed leaves, eggs, yogurt, and human cell samples. He has found, for example, that white cells taken from a person's mouth and placed in a test tube still respond electrochemically to the donor's emotional states, even when the donor is out of the room, out of the building, or out of the state (keep this in mind for the next chapter!).

His experiments with plants included hooking them up with electrodes to a lie detector, which registered every "emotional reaction" they had, especially to traumatic events. They didn't have to be involved "personally." They reacted even when shrimp was dropped in boiling water several rooms away or hot water was going down the sink—which hurt the live bacteria in it.

In similar experiments, trees that were monitored showed no reaction until other trees in the vicinity were being cut down by a lumberjack. The next day they demonstrated violent reactions as soon as the lumberjack showed up!

Isn't it great how we can draw a parallel between the Masaru Emoto's work with water and Cleve Backster's work with plants?

In quantum physics similar theories claim that not only plants but every individual atom has a certain consciousness. This means that, in theory, we could energetically affect anyone and anything—period!

It is important to note that when working with large plants that are too big for our embrace or close-up treatment, we have to expand our "vision" and type of treatment. The previously noted large oak tree would be really hard to treat just standing next to it in the usual way. In this case, more visualizing is necessary, as well as a more open mind (not that your mind hasn't opened by now!). One way of working on a colossal tree is to picture your energy coming out of your hands being much larger or, better yet, longer. See your energy expanding to not only several feet wide but even hundreds of yards, if necessary. You will be surprised by how far you will be able to feel a tree's energy. Your hands will pick up the imbalances just like working with a person next to you. The distance doesn't matter! As a matter of fact, distance is an obstacle only to a limited mind. When you close your eyes, how long does it take you to think of a familiar place and be there (in your mind only—of course)? A millisecond maybe? In the case of the tree standing in front of you, you don't even have to close your eyes. There is not much to visualize at all, just the energy leaving your hands. True visualization is needed only if the subject of your energy healing is farther than your sight distance. For that purpose, you better learn long-distance healing.

15.
Long-Distance
Healing

Long-distance healing (LDH) or Distance Healing is the ability to heal someone who is not in your presence. We know by now that we can work on individuals without touching them. We can do that from several inches away, several feet away, several miles away, or even continents away. Remember the experience of thinking of someone—just before the phone rings with that person on the other line?

All radio waves are invisible, yet they reach incredible distances. Since our minds also produce frequencies, it shouldn't be hard to grasp this concept.

There are several theories on how long-distance healing—or telepathy for that matter—works, but there is still no firm evidence in existence. This is similar to how we know a lot about the human energy field, but nobody can really measure it with modern instruments. We know about many scientific tests about telepathy, including the ones performed by the military, but the results are deemed inconclusive.

There were many experiments on the power of prayer—when groups of individuals pray for certain people they have never met.

Those also ended with confusing outcomes. It worked for some while it didn't for others. There was not enough evidence to draw a scientific conclusion.

Some hypothesize that the earth's frequency, which is somewhere close to 12 Hz, may carry our mind's frequency, which is in the same neighborhood when we are in the alpha state of meditation or daydreaming. Others postulate that it is the higher frequencies we produce that penetrate everything and travel distances. It is up to science to discover the truth.

Disregarding what science has to say at the given moment, I have been performing long-distance healing for more than two decades with positive results. I can't claim that it works for everyone—just like regular bioenergy healing doesn't work for everyone either. However, the evidence so far (and all the satisfied customers) implies that it makes a difference indeed.

Some teachers will tell you to become proficient in energy healing in person before ever attempting long-distance healing, but I disagree. The energy doesn't recognize any distance; it is limited only by our minds. I believe that it is important to develop our visualization from the very beginning. What better way to do it than to work on someone who is not in your presence. Some of you have excellent abilities to visualize and have a wild imagination. Others, a bit less. For that reason, we will start from scratch.

There are several ways to perform LDH, of which I will teach you my favorites. They all require some proficiency in meditation. For beginners, I recommend Jose Silva's Mind Control, but there are many other good choices as well. I use a combination of several methods with some additions from my own experiences. If you have never meditated before, a good ability to daydream is a sufficient start. Nevertheless, let's learn some basics.

Contrary to general belief, you don't just end up at a blissful place of no thoughts when you meditate—unless you have some incredible abilities honed over many decades of self-deprivation and an egoless existence. For us mere mortals, that is a very far place. We have quite a hard time just shutting up the chatter in our minds—not necessarily crazy voices but our own everyday thoughts. Think about it: is there a moment in your day when you don't hear the voice? It is your own, but nevertheless, it is a voice in your head. Sometimes it comes in a form of a song that you can't get out of your mind. Sometimes it is just you thinking of what you have to do next. Sometimes it is gibberish. It is a busy place, the mind. The meditation objective of a regular human is to focus all thoughts and chatter into one. If we can concentrate on only one thing, our brain can take a nice break from everything else. That is incidentally an added benefit of LDH—while you work on someone, your brain is actually resting from everyday problems and the pressures of the "real" world.

Let's start with a basic relaxation technique for the body.

Sit or lie down in a quiet comfortable setting. Make sure that there are no distractions of any kind. Breathe deeply yet at ease. Now concentrate on your feet. You may tighten them up to focus your thoughts even more on them. While they are tight, take a deep breath. As you exhale, relax your feet and forget about them. Focus your attention on your calves now. Tighten them up as you take a deep breath, and relax them as you exhale. Forget about them as well. Next step is the upper legs. Then come the buttocks, followed by the back, the shoulders, arms, hands, stomach, and neck. Use the same system for the entire body, finishing with the facial muscles. Lastly, take a few deep yet relaxed breaths as you focus on only your breathing. By now, your heart rate should be slow and relaxed as well. Stay in that relaxed state, concentrating on only your breathing. You are in the moment now. Nothing else exists for you but your breath.

Now let's focus on the mind.

In order to remove your attention from the body altogether, focus on your eyes. While they stay shut, look up at the area between your eyebrows (a.k.a. the third eye), as if you were inside your own head looking out. You may feel a bit of tension or tingling there. All you will see is black or dark purple. Stay there for a moment.

Now focus on seeing numbers. Count down from ten to one while taking a deep (and still relaxed) breath for each number. You should see them in white. If you have a hard time imagining these, try to visualize them being written on a blackboard, like in school. One breath, one number, slowly counting down. With each number you will be more relaxed and more focused. Once you reach number one, you will let go entirely. There will be no more body. You will be deep in your mind. This is a perfect place for relaxation. It is also the perfect place for long-distance healing.

At this point you start the actual meditation with a purpose.

Visualize a place of serenity. It can be anywhere on the planet or beyond. It should also be a place where you can perform your work at ease. In my mind, I prefer the inside of a pyramid. I used it long before I had the privilege to be inside several of them. However, you can choose any other place you are comfortable with. It can be a familiar place or something totally out of your imagination. You can set it up as an office (with a computer, clock, calendar—in case you need those for your sessions) or just keep it natural and outdoorsy if you wish. It is helpful if this place has a screen, such as a movie screen as a background. It aids the visualization process. Some people actually like to set up their special place in a movie theatre for an easier mental picture.

You will start with some simple visualization exercises. Make one side of the screen an entrance and the other an exit. You will bring in your subjects from the entrance and let them out through the exit when you are done with them. For starters, let's concentrate on something you are quite familiar with. Bring in an apple, and place it in front of the screen. You should have it hover in front of the screen, thus giving you the full 3D visual. Examine it carefully. See the color, the shape, the texture. See it up close. You may hold it in your hand if you wish (still in your mind only of course). You have to know that you can do anything in your mind. For starters, however, do things that you can do in real life, such as slice the apple in half. Examine it carefully and up close. See the inside texture, the seeds, the chamber holding the seeds, the little veins, the thin skin. After you are done with all the little details and you can see everything vividly, you may put the apple back together. Look at it one more time, and let it off toward the exit. You may repeat this exercise with other fruits and vegetables. Any citrus fruit in particular can give a vivid impression to the point of affecting your salivary glands when you imagine peeling the fruit, smelling it, or drinking the juice. Practice this for several days until you feel that you are proficient in it.

When done, bring your focus back to numbers. You may see them on the same movie screen that you just created. You may even see them as if they were at the beginning of an old film reel, with circles appearing around them. This time count up from one to ten. One breath, one number! As your count climbs upward, so does your awareness. For the last few numbers, concentrate more on your breathing. By number ten, you will be aware of your surroundings and your own self. You will feel relaxed, refreshed, content, and back in reality.

Now you are ready for people.

Following the previously described routine, get to the same comfortable state of body and mind that you have established. You can probably do it faster by now. At a later point, you may group together some body parts or skip that part entirely and focus on the mind. You may not even need to concentrate on relaxing your body any more. You can also reduce the numbers that you count from ten to maybe only five. Potentially, you can arrive at your alpha state within seconds.

Choose people with whom you are very familiar as the first few people you work with. You ought to know them well enough to be able to visualize their features, especially their faces. They don't have to be aware of you working on them, unless you would like feedback. In that case, make sure that they know the exact time of the treatment, for which they should lie down or sit still with their eyes shut. You may tell them to start before you, so they are relaxed by the time you start your work. They should stay in that position for at least half an hour. Many of them will feel the session as if you were in their presence.

Go through your routine, and get settled in your special place/office/movie theatre. Look up at the screen, and make sure that you see it clearly. Now bring in the person you wish to work on to the middle of the screen (again from the side of the screen that you established as an entrance). Look at their silhouette first, and then get closer where you can recognize their features (keep in mind that you can do anything in your imagination—move them far, close, turn them around, and even look inside them). Look at the face, and examine every little detail, as if the person was right there in front of you. When clear, look at the rest of the body. Now step away slightly, and try to see the energy around them. This will take a little practice and definitely some trust in your abilities. "The first thought is the best," a card player would say. This may take some time. Don't stress about it. When you think you can see the energy, you probably do see it. Examine every detail of it—the thickness, the lightness, the irregularity. Can you see darker areas in it? Can you see where it is too thick or too thin? If you do, you may proceed with the treatment based on those observations. Again, no stress if you can't see any of that. In that case, you can proceed with the treatment based on the subject's comments (or medical diagnoses) alone.

As I mentioned before, there are several different treatment methods.

In the **first one** you proceed exactly the way you would in a real one-on-one session. Except, in this case, you would do it in your mind alone. Can't visualize your hand moves? No problem! Move your hands for real while your eyes are still shut. You may even feel the familiar tension, heat, and tingling as in an "actual" treatment. One day when you are better at visualizing, you can let the hands relax and have the brain do the work. Quite frankly, the better you can visualize (and the deeper you are in meditative state), the better the LDH will work.

At a higher level of this practice, you don't have to stop at the energy field. You can take a peek inside the body as well. As a matter of fact, you can examine every organ and even (if you really take your time!) every cell if you wish. You can perform energetic surgery and remove the "bad" energy at will. It helps the visualization process if you have already established what the "bad" or excess energy looks like. Most people see it as hazy, dark gray or even black at the worst areas. In your mind, you can grab those, and pull them out of the field, replacing them with white or clean energy. In case of tumors, you can visualize pulling all the dark energy out and strengthening the surrounding area with pure white energy. Or if you can imagine it, pull the entire tumor out, and refill the area with the healthy white substance.

When you are done working on someone, you may want to visualize the full, healthy energy field around them as a white glow in the exact size the field should be (an arm's-length wide).

This brings us to the **second method of LDH.** In this technique you just visualize the energy of the person and simply clean the dirty, gray, dark or black areas and replace them with the clean white energy. It doesn't sound very scientific, but by now your brain has established the difference between good and bad, and it will automatically associate those colors and shades with the energy. It will take some time before you get to this level, but once here, it makes healing very simple and effective.

Either method you use, when done with your subject, you may escort them off the stage toward the pre-established exit. You may even place them in a relaxing lounge area if you wish. If you want to add some additional blessings, white light, direct connection to heaven, or anything else that you deem necessary, go ahead and do it. There is nothing you can't do. It is all up to your imagination.

Several years ago, a good friend of mine, who is a working medium, was visiting London and was suffering from a bad cold that nearly knocked her down. She had a debilitating headache, pressure in her sinuses and difficulty breathing—all of that happening the day before her scheduled presentation to a large audience. In her desperation, she called me up in the middle of the night (it was late evening in my time zone) and asked if I could work on her. I immediately sat down and went into a deep meditation. I concentrated fully on the energy itself and removed all the dark haziness from her sinus areas, her head, and her lungs. I replaced them all with pure white energy and made sure that her field was as wide as it should be. I engulfed her in a pure white glow. I saw her exceptionally vividly, a lot more than usual. She called me up the next day to thank me profusely and to tell me that she was doing great.

A few months later I was attending one of her lectures. She brought up this experience to her audience and sheepishly admitted that, in the middle of the night when I worked on her, she saw a vision of me appearing at the foot of her bed. I was smiling, and I was all in white!

Some practitioners like to have helpers with them. You can visualize anyone you want, dead or alive, to help you in your healing. It can be a famous healer, doctor, or anyone from your family or friends whom you think would provide some comfort or actual assistance in your endeavors. You can have them sit or stand beside or behind you. They don't really have to do anything, but their presence alone may be a help to you. Use your imagination!

I have to mention another method that I use sporadically, when my brain is not 100 percent there. Let's call this the **Breath LDH** technique. It is very helpful in those very rare occasions when I may be too busy, have too much on my mind, or there is some kind of family chaos around me that won't let me concentrate fully. When your mind starts doing tricks on you, it may be elsewhere, ahead of time (planning to take the car to get serviced, etc.), back in time (forgot to pick up the car), or similarly distracted. Concentrating on your breathing brings you back, but sometimes that is not enough. Your thoughts may wander again. In that case, I combine the two: I concentrate on my breathing while working on someone. When I already have my subject in my view, I take a deep yet relaxed breath, and I move the energy as I exhale. I repeat that for each body part. Inhale at the head, exhale as I pull the excess energy away, and throw it away. Inhale at the neck, exhale as I throw the energy away, and so on. Once the energy field is clear, I can do the opposite: inhale and, as I exhale, refill the entire energy field with the fresh, clean, white healing energy. Usually by the time I am done with my first client, I am already in the zone and in the moment, so I don't have to concentrate on my breathing for the next person I work on. Some energy healing methods use a similar breathing during the whole time. You may try it in a regular one-on-one treatment as well.

When working on someone that I have never met, I find it helpful to know their name (it's a must!), age, and approximate location (New York City, Los Angeles, Sidney). A recent photo of the person is more than supportive. Pictures, as we know, carry the energy of the person; thus it takes less effort to imagine them. However, the healing still works if there is no picture at all.

I ask my clients if they care when I work on them or if they want to actually feel the treatment at a predetermined time. Quite frankly, it is not necessary for them to concentrate on the treatments at all. They can go ahead with their usual days, and the healing will still work. As a matter of fact, I get strange requests sometimes, including a common one in which someone (usually a woman) asks if I can work on a spouse (usually a man) without the spouse's knowledge— "Because they don't believe in this stuff" is the usual explanation.

The answer is, of course, yes. Just as you can work on animals and babies, who especially have no idea you are working on them, you can work on anyone without his/her knowledge. There is no belief factor involved, so it is energy healing in its purest form.

Most of my clients, however, love to feel the treatments. I set a time with them, and while I meditate and do the LDH, they lie down or sit still with their eyes closed and enjoy the treatment. Most of them feel the exact sensations as if I were right there doing it personally. They feel the tingling, the movement of the energy, the heat, sometimes cold, when I pull the energy off—and all the other feelings that come with healing. Many times there are incredible and unusual effects and side effects as well.

Here is a testimonial from a sixty-six-year-old woman:

> *"During the session, my back usually first elongates, then left/right side shifts until right neck and shoulder relax and release. Last time, I could feel energy at my third eye too. Afterward, I felt good. I have more sexual energy and even had an orgasm in my dream which has never happened in a dream before!"*

Several years ago, I discovered that I could work on others even without closing my eyes or meditating per se. I can even do it while driving (don't try this at home, kids!)! It is a form of daydreaming that allows this, requiring only a part of the brain while the other part still performs your daily tasks. It is good for emergencies, I guess, but for real healing you do have to meditate.

In a similar fashion, **instant LDH** happens at the highest level of your development. There is a point that you can reach where your mind is so open and so focused that you don't have to go through any of the previous exercises to be in the presence of your subject. You can just think of them, see them, and see them completely healthy all in an instant. As soon as you perceive the perfectly healthy energy in and around them, the healing is complete. If you can do all of the above in a few seconds, you have achieved instant long-distance healing. Keep practicing, and it will become a regular occurrence.

I have a regular client who I see twice a month. Every time I work on her, her little dog comes between us and starts making faces. He turns his head sideways and pays close attention to the energy as if he wanted part of the action. I may give him a quick pat on his head, but I generally ignore him. He just seems very happy with the surrounding energy. This only happens during the healing session. If we just stand and talk, he stays away and is totally uninterested. He only comes between us when the energy flows. One day, my client called with a headache and wondered if I could do some quick long-distance work on her. It was my lunch hour, so I just closed my eyes and started working on her right there in the restaurant. As I performed the LDH, she told me later, her dog started acting strangely and proceeded with his usual faces at the usual spot, except that now he was at a loss because I wasn't there! I have heard of similar experiences from other clients as well. If you need validation of LDH, ask the pets!

Here are a few more recent LDH testimonials and observations from around the world (some are still in ongoing treatment, just to illustrate the feedback I get from my clients):

"Thanks. There is a marked improvement in the headaches. I'm very happy and at the same time almost afraid to hope that they're finally going to be a thing of the past."

"A note to let you know it was another amazing session today! :) I feel wonderful :) About ten minutes into the session I felt a slight (but distinct) heaviness in the heart region of my chest. Within a few seconds that completely disappeared and that entire region felt very light :) It was a wonderful feeling, and a very distinct feeling that something 'released.' That's the only way I know to describe it."

"Heart rate and breathing have been great since I last contacted you. Thanks for your hard work (and gifted work!). I truly appreciate it."

"As far as my mom, she has been feeling much much better. She has been in consistent good health ever since you started working on her. Her mild headaches are gone since last week Wednesday."

"Getting ahead of the game today to tell you about the session just now. My cat came into my lap as soon as I sat down, which is usual, but he immediately began to purr and then snore. I felt your energy moving through my feet up to my head but more quickly until I felt all full and then something like weak, as if a lot was loosened at once. I quickly fell asleep in the chair! Could hardly wake, really, and am now lying on a heating mat, unable to do much. Still feel a thickness in my head. And a tingling through my body. I feel great!"

"Thank you! Josh is doing great. He hasn't had to use any of his allergy medicine for several weeks. Another treatment three weeks from now sounds good. I'll keep up the neck exercises. Have a great weekend!"

"My leg was much better after your work last week so if you could do another session tomorrow that would be great."

"Hi Csongor,
Thanks for the session.
My blood results have arrived and most of them are really positive.
My insomnia has improved in the last few days, so that is good as well!"

"Thank you VERY much for all of the work you've done to help me. There are not enough words to express my gratitude. I'm very thankful for you and your gift of healing, and your patience in giving me updates and answering my questions. Many many thanks to you."

"My lung pain left five mins after your treatment. Thank you!!!! Felt like a tow truck on my chest before!!!"

"I know you will be doing distance healing for my mom tomorrow but you don't have to include my son again. After last week's session he is doing much better. His cough almost stopped that evening when you did the healing and he has recovered a lot since. Thank you for your help."

"Yes . . . I really felt the power again today . . . I was even vibrating for a few seconds from top to bottom, sitting in the chair. I do feel significantly better, and have begun to leave off my knee support with no pain resulting.
Thank you!!!"

Bonus
Chapters

Dowsing Overview

Ever since you were born, certain signals became embedded in your subconscious. They were divided into positive and negative groups. From the earliest age of simple signals (stomach ache = bad/ negative; mother's milk = good/positive) to the more complicated signs of adulthood (subtle electromagnetic fields, other people's moods, etc.), our subconscious became the decision maker on the yin and yang of our being. We have certain reactions to everything around us. However, we may not always be able to read the subtle messages that come with those. The subconscious is connected to the entire universe, yet we hardly ever tap into that knowledge. There are exceptions, such as the ones that we already mentioned (phone ringing when we think of a certain person, stopping before an accident, picking the right route, etc.), but they usually come on their own, out of our control. There are a few ways to tap into that universal knowledge. Meditation is one of them, but it is limited to time and mind. Kinesiology (muscle testing) is a good source of tapping into the subconscious, but unless you are an exceptional master, you need a partner to do the testing on.

Dowsing can be the shortest and fastest way to a solo subconscious trip. It brings out the positive or negative answer to any question within seconds. Our bodies are already the instruments; we just need the indicator that shows the answers. That's where dowsing tools come into play.

Have you ever seen or heard of people looking for underground water with the help of a couple of rods, or just a twig? Have you heard of oil companies employing individuals with special gifts to look for underground oil with the help of a simple pendulum? Those are certainly not scientific instruments but are up to the task.

More than 80 percent of people are able to perform dowsing the first time they try it. Why should *you* learn it? Answer: When you run into a problem that you can't figure out or need to pinpoint a negative area in the body or find negative areas in a house that affect someone's health, dowsing is a powerful assistant. Since there are dozens of excellent books on the subject, we will just cover the basics.

First of all, you need the aforementioned indicator for your instrument. Let's skip the twig, and go straight to a pendulum. Anything that you can hang on a string can become a pendulum. For your personal instrument, you should start with a small weight, such as a bead or a machine nut (8mm is the best) that you would tie to a thin string or thread. Make the length of the string 8–12 inches, and tie a knot on it about 5–6 inches from

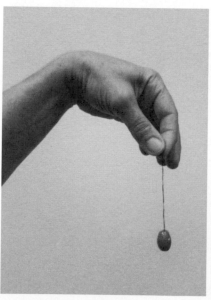
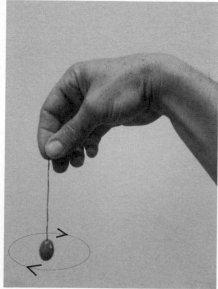

the bead. Your instrument is complete! You may also purchase a dowsing tool. There is quite a selection out there. Some people prefer fancy, jewel-like pendulums with crystals hanging on them while others like the precise feel of good electrical conductors such as brass, silver, or gold. The rounded ones may be comfortable in your pocket while the pointy ends of some others help with more precise work—over maps, for instance.

To use your new instrument, all you have to do is hold the knot on the string between your thumb and forefinger (with your palm facing down) and let your hand relax. Now, either out loud or in your head, repeat the word "yes." This is a positive word that will bring out the positive reaction in your body. The pendulum will start spinning either clockwise or counterclockwise. Whichever way it goes, that is your "yes." Now, think or say "no" repeatedly. The pendulum will swing out and spin the opposite way. That is your "no" answer. Those directions will never change in your lifetime. Now, you have the open connection with your subconscious. All you have to do is ask questions that can be answered by "yes" or "no"!

Example

"Is there negative energy in this room?" If yes, "Is there more than one spot of negative energy in this room?" If yes, you can explore further by asking if the number is between one and five or more than five and so on. You may ask which direction the negative energy is in. In that case, the pendulum will swing out toward the negative energy instead of spinning around. Once you have the direction, you should change your position in the room, and ask the question again to get the exact mark (see p. 224). The opportunities and combinations are endless.

The most important thing in dowsing is that you have to be a neutral party in order to get the right answer. If you are emotionally involved, your answers will reflect your conscious mind, which may not know the actual truth. For instance, if you were asking questions

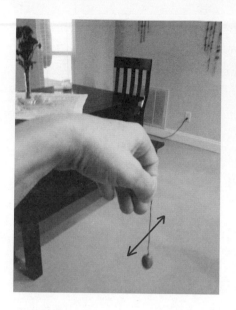 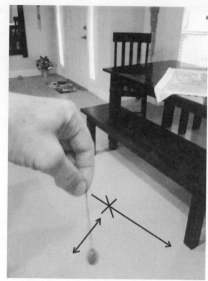

about your mom's or child's health, it will show you that everything is okay, just because that is your conscious wish. Neutrality guarantees success. (That may be the reason no one has hit the lottery jackpot with the help of dowsing!)

Whatever you decide to do with this knowledge, please do adequate practicing before you apply it in the real world. You can practice in a form of a game with friends and family. Look for an object that someone hid from you: have a friend mix up a few cards, and find the one red card among the blacks while they are face down, or other such games. Your subconscious will be on fire!

In the bioenergy world, you may ask the pendulum how many times you may have to treat someone in order for the energy to stay in balance. Or ask how many minutes you have to energize, how often, and so on. There is an answer to every question if you ask it right.

If the question is number-related, you may draw yourself a percentage diagram (or copy the one on p. 225). Here you would hold the pendulum over the center of the diagram and ask the question "how many . . . ?" to get your answer. The pendulum will

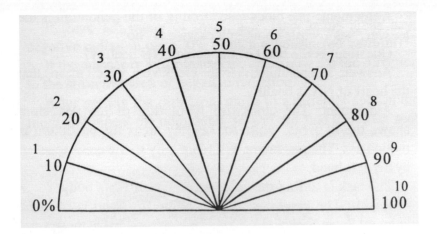

swing out in the direction of the right number. If the answer is off the scale or if the question is not right, the pendulum will spin around. For instance: how many imbalances are there in this person's body? The pendulum will swing out to number 3 if there are that many imbalances. However, if there are more than 10, it won't be able to answer you. In that case you would ask: how many imbalances over 10?

As you can tell, the scale has two sets of numbers. One row shows percentages from 0 to 100, while the second row shows numbers from 0 to 10. The combination of these can answer any number related question. Keep practicing!

When looking for negative areas, don't be surprised if they are caused by everyday items that you previously never thought harmful. Negativity can come from anywhere, anything, and anyone.

Some twenty years ago I was asked to work on a friend's baby. She had a hard time falling asleep and staying asleep. The parents were desperate. They noticed that when they were visiting family and friends, the baby slept better at their houses than at home. That gave me a hint that maybe they put the baby in a negative area. Babies, just like animals, are very sensitive to energy fields. While animals can stay away from negative areas (dogs will never lie in a negative spot), babies are stuck where we put them.

I checked the bedroom where the crib was located and couldn't find one positive area. Even the old grandfather clock was negative, not to mention the TV set. After checking the rest of the house, I concluded that the only positive spot for the crib was situated in a corner of the kitchen/dining room. Reluctantly, the parents positioned the crib in that spot, and lo and behold, the baby fell asleep. I left it to them to explain to their visitors why the baby lived in the kitchen, but everyone was happy nevertheless!

I still use my pendulum from time to time when I get stuck with certain clients who don't react to the healing or go back to the same imbalances soon after their sessions. In those cases, I would look at the energy of their homes or workplaces to try to find the source of their distress. You may want to do the same.

Healthy Living Overview

If you want to become an exceptionally good healer, you have to be in exceptionally good health yourself. Just as you wouldn't go to a mechanic whose car is falling apart or you wouldn't hire a personal trainer who is out of shape, you shouldn't expect people to ask for your help if you are sick yourself. It is not only about appearances. In order for the energy to freely flow through you, your energy field should be in perfect health. You cannot give others your own illness or problem. On the other hand, when you are healthy, your own energy keeps replenishing and refreshing itself every time you work on someone else. Thus, the more you work on others, the more you work on yourself. Quite a bonus, isn't it? However, energy healing itself is not enough. There are many factors that affect your health, which we have already mentioned in the chapter on the reasons for illness. You have to address all of them in order to be healthy. Mind, body, spirit—they all need maintenance every day of your life. Modern technology provides answers to every question at the push of a button. Please utilize it if you have any questions. You have to educate yourself constantly since new discoveries happen as we speak. Remember when smoking was okay? Or when fat was bad? We know that sugar is public enemy number one, but what about other things that are still unknown to the public? A keen eye to new research is essential to your health and to the health of your clients.

A Healthy Body

It would be impossible to list everything required for a healthy body. There are some things that we can't help, such as our genes or maybe even our surroundings (if it is impossible for us to move). However, there are many things that we can do. I will list just a few that are very important.

Healthy diet

- Mostly alkaline foods (close to 4/5 of your diet), packed with fresh organic vegetables, fruit, nuts, seeds, green juices, smoothies, and such
- Wholesome food, nothing processed—as close to its natural state as possible
- If unable to get it from food itself, additional supplements of minerals and vitamins
- Five to six meals a day, none so big as to overwhelm the body (too much food all at once, especially meat and other acidic foods, will take away energy from the rest of the body that is needed to digest). A meal compressed to the size of your fist is adequate to fill your stomach without stretching it. Stop eating when you feel 80 percent full.
- Lots of water (clean, alkaline). I have to remind you here that water takes in energy very easily. Why not energize it before drinking it? Hold your energy ball (with tight fingers) over the water or around your glass for a few seconds and voila: you have energized water! Or just be nice to it—think of Emoto.
- Before you eat the meal in front of you, you may want to give thanks for (to) it. This doesn't have to be based on a

religious reason. You may give thanks to the universe, the persons who harvested your food, the ones who prepared it, or to all and everything at once. Just give thanks—the positive energy will reinforce the already existing energy in the food itself.

The food pyramid has been replaced by the food circle. The guidelines have changed and are still changing!

Healthy exercise

- Not all exercises fit every individual. Find what is adequate for your age and abilities. However, everyone needs some cardiovascular exercise, strength training, and stretching. Some exercises such as yoga, t'ai chi, and qigong have additional benefits to your energy field. I have found that a combination of different disciplines works best for me. I train with weights three times a week; fast-walk every day for at least half an hour; run, bike, or swim once a week for at least half an hour; do yoga once a week for at least an hour to an hour and a half; and practice t'ai chi and QiGong at least twice a week for half an hour. In addition, I don't start my day without my stretching and energizing routine (see p. 232).

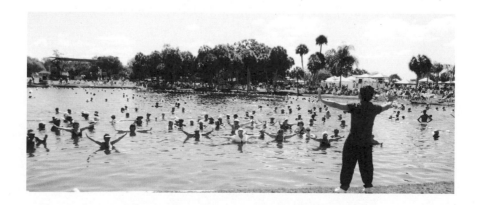

- If you have no experience in exercise, try joining a club or a yoga studio, and follow the instructions of an experienced practitioner.
- The most important exercise of them all:

Even if you are the laziest person on the planet, you can still take a couple of minutes a day to perform a qigong swing. This is a must for everyone! I call it **The Ultimate Energy-Enhancing Exercise.** It is one of the simplest yet most incredible exercises that have ever been developed. Its variations have been practiced in China for centuries and are credited for rewarding the practitioner with health and youthful vigor.

The Ultimate Energy-Enhancing Exercise

*The basic **swing** is performed in a standing position with your feet shoulder width apart, knees slightly bent and your pelvis tucked under. Your upper body should be straight, head up. Make sure your arms are totally relaxed like a pair of wet noodles hanging by your sides. Turn to one side, and let your body's flexibility pull you back toward the middle. Since your arms are relaxed, your body will turn a bit past the middle. Let it go and let your arms go a little farther. With just a little bit added energy, your body will now turn the opposite direction. As you continue this, after a while, you will be turning effortlessly left and right. As you speed up, you will turn farther and farther, increasing the stretching and twisting in your spine and in the entire body. Try to look behind you at every turn and let your arms slap you both in the back and in the front.*

The twisting will move every vertebra (even if some of them will move only microscopically); it will stretch not only your neck and back muscles,

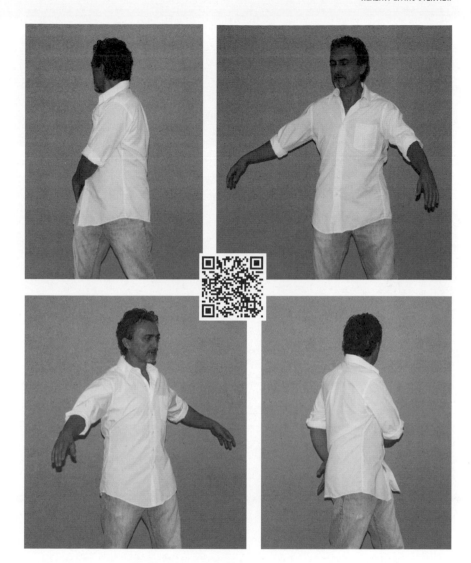

but the entire body all the way down to your toes. Your fascia (the sheets encapsulating the muscles) will stretch as well. Your shoulders will try to separate due to the centripetal power pulling them outside—this will create a vacuum in your shoulder joints, pulling in more lubrication. Your blood circulation will increase, especially to your

233

hands. Your lymph circulation will be encouraged as well. The energy will be forced through the body almost like when you heal, thus improving your energy flow, too. The slapping will massage your internal organs, improving their function as an additional bonus. The list of all the benefits is very long. Again, even if you claim that you have no time at all, you can always borrow a few minutes from your busy day for your own benefit.

- The absolute best exercise for your energy, your cardiovascular system, and a clear mind is making love. It does feel good for a reason!

For those enthusiastic to have a good start for the day and to help prevent injuries, as well as to get energized, here is my morning routine. It takes only five to ten minutes (I usually do it during my morning dog walk while he is sniffing around):

- **Empty stance:** Stand up with your feet parallel, shoulder width apart, knees slightly bent, with your pelvis tucked under. The upper body should be straight, head up, shoulders relaxed. This is also a good posture if you have to stand for a very long time.
- **Neck roll:** Slowly drop your head forward, so your chin touches your chest. Gently roll your head left and right, while trying to keep the chin on the chest. Go farther with each turn, until you reach your shoulder with your ear after about ten rolls. Don't worry if they don't touch—they can't if you are keeping your shoulders down. Now continue to roll your head all the way around. Ten times one way, ten times the other. Try not to turn your head—just roll. This will stretch and warm your neck and shoulders as well as open the neck passages for good energy flow.

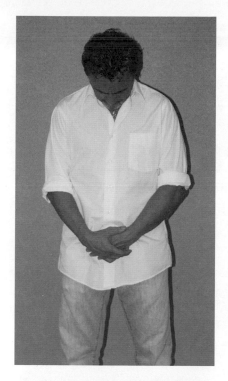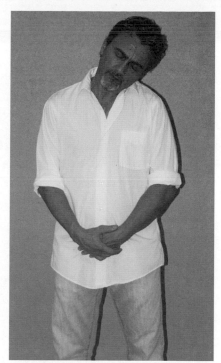

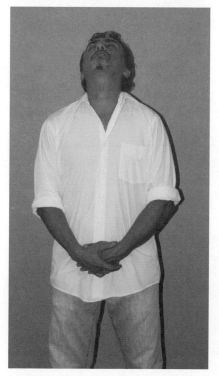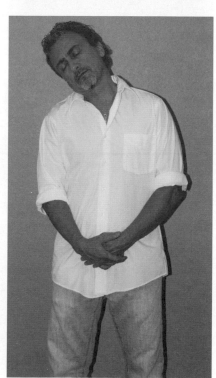

- **Shoulder roll:** Lift your arms up sideways, so they are the same height as your shoulders. Point your palms away from your body, and pull your fingers back as far as possible. Now start circling your arms first backward ten times and then forward ten times, gradually increasing the diameter of the circles. Follow that by turning your hands down (palms facing you this time) and doing ten large circles both back and forward. This will warm up your shoulders and arms as well as stretch them, especially the forearms. Energy will be coming to your hands!

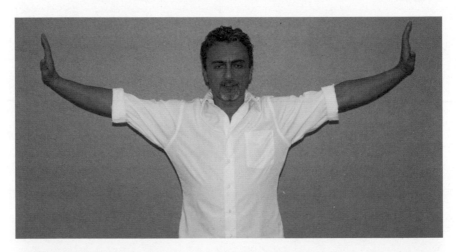

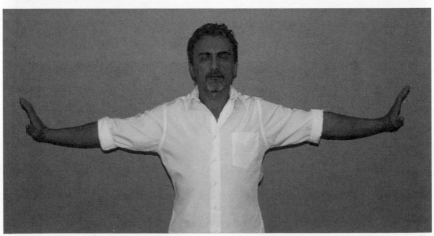

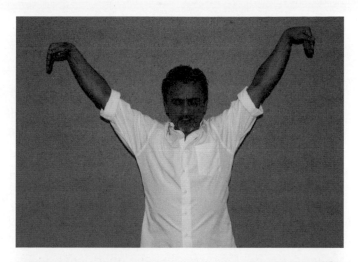

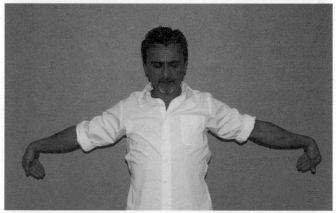

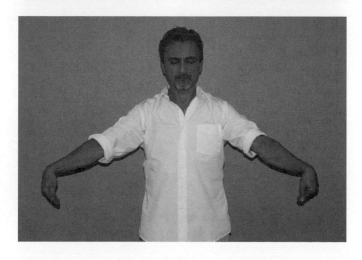

- **Hugs:** As soon as you stop circling your arms, start giving yourself dynamic hugs. Stretch your arms back as far as they go shoulder height, and then slap yourself forward with both arms as they cross one over the other across the chest. Repeat ten times. This is a good stretch for the shoulders as well as a good stimulant for the energy flow down the arms.
- **Swing:** The ultimate energy-enhancing exercise (see p. 230).
- **Quad stretch:** Pull your right foot up behind your buttocks with your right hand and hold for ten seconds while tucking under the pelvis. Repeat on the left. If you are unable to do this, hold onto something solid (like a tree), and squat down for ten seconds. This stretches the quadriceps and sends the energy down the knees.

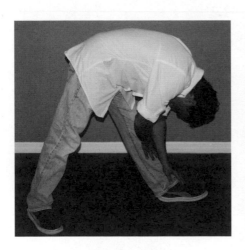

Hamstring stretch

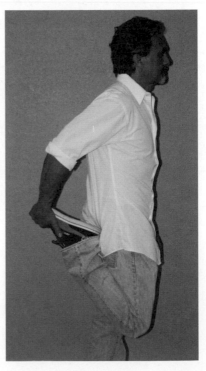

Quad stretch

- **Hamstring stretch:** Step out straight with the left foot about two feet in front of the right, which is turned out 45 degrees. With both knees straight and the hips turned forward, slowly exhale and lower your upper body gently over the front leg. You will feel a nice stretch in your left hamstring. Hold for ten seconds, and repeat on the other side. This will stretch the lower back as well and open the energy passages down to your feet.
- **Foot roll:** Standing on one foot, lift the other behind onto your toes and circle ten times. Repeat on the other foot. This will loosen and warm your ankles, letting the energy flow through them easier.
- In addition, if you are in a good shape I would also recommend the **Sun Salutation** from any yoga routine.

If you have thirty-five to forty-five minutes a day that you would like to devote to energy-enhancing exercises, I would highly recommend *Energizing t'ai chi Chi Kung*—a double DVD set by yours truly—available on www.csongordaniel.com.

A healthy mind

Your mind needs daily exercise just like your body. "If you don't use it, you lose it" is a rule for your mind, too. The mind is the main source of your happiness or sadness, relaxation or stress. Having a positive attitude certainly helps, but there is a lot more to keeping a healthy mind. Please read up on mindfulness, being in the now, and letting go of the ego. Meditation is a great source of a healthy, stress-free mind.

In addition:

- Reread chapter 4 on positive thinking.
- Play chess, checkers, cards, or any other social game where you are challenged by others (and you socialize as well!).

- Meet with friends, family, and interesting people as much as possible.
- Read books and solve crossword puzzles.
- Get to the bottom of mechanical problems.
- Learn a new language.
- Satisfy your curiosity!
- Be in love!
- Be kind!

The healthy spirit

Wherever you come from, your spiritual health is very important. If you are religious, it may mean daily prayers, going to church weekly, or participating in any other form of worship. You can have a healthy spirit even if you are not affiliated with any religion. The important thing is to believe. The source of your belief may not even be as important as the fact itself that you believe (okay, if you believe in your pastrami sandwich or some evil cult, that may not work). One of the best exercises that you can do is give daily thanks to all the good things around you: your food, family, shelter, job, friends, and countless other blessings. You may even want to write down a list of positive things around you and keep it in plain view either on your bathroom mirror or the refrigerator. Add to the inventory every day. There is never an end to that list, and it will keep your positive things in perspective. The energy is all around you and permeates everything. Whatever messages you send out to the universe will come back to you even more enhanced as if under the control of an infinitive powerful magnet.

It is important to know that there is more to life than what we see. There is a higher purpose to everything. We are part of that higher purpose; thus our actions contribute to the betterment of the universe.

About the Author

Csongor Daniel has more than a quarter of a century's experience in bioenergy healing. Starting with a gift but no healing knowledge while an engineering student at the age of 21, he went through the full spectrum of education, from self-learning to studying with one of the world's foremost healers, Zdenko Domancic. Fresh out of college, he managed to work on 30 people a day within the first three months of his practice.

In the United States since 1991, Csongor (pronounced Chongor) has published two books on bioenergy healing and a t'ai chi double DVD set to share his knowledge. His acclaimed light and humorous lectures, both in the states and internationally, continue to expand the number of his followers and the advocates of this simple yet powerful healing method.

Csongor's books and videos as well as online lectures are available at www.csongordaniel.com.